Short-Term
Dynamic Psychotherapy

Evaluation and Technique

SECOND EDITION

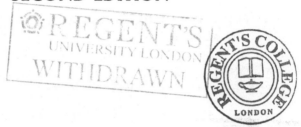

TOPICS IN GENERAL PSYCHIATRY

Series Editor:

John C. Nemiah, M.D.
*Professor of Psychiatry, Dartmouth Medical School
and Professor of Psychiatry Emeritus, Harvard Medical School*

Short-Term Dynamic Psychotherapy

Evaluation and Technique

SECOND EDITION

Peter E. Sifneos, M.D.

Harvard Medical School
Boston, Massachusetts

PLENUM MEDICAL BOOK COMPANY
NEW YORK AND LONDON

Library of Congress Cataloging in Publication Data

Sifneos, Peter E. (Peter Emmanuel), 1920–
  Short-term dynamic psychotherapy.

  (Topics in general psychiatry)
  Bibliography: p.
  Includes index.
  1. Psychotherapy, Brief. 2. Anxiety. I. Title. II. Series. [DNLM: 1. Anxiety. 2. Inter-
view, Psychological. 3. Psychotherapy, Brief. WM 420 S573sb]
RC480.55.S55   1987   616.89'14   87-2346
ISBN 0-306-42341-3

First Printing—May 1987
Second Printing—February 1990

© 1987 Plenum Publishing Corporation
233 Spring Street, New York, N.Y. 10013

Plenum Medical Book Company is an imprint of Plenum Publishing Corporation

TO JEANNETTE

Understanding and warm
Tolerant and magnanimous
A tower of strength
A beloved sister

Foreword to the Second Edition

In the seven years since Dr. Sifneos's *Short-Term Dynamic Psychotherapy* first appeared, it has become one of the classic works on the subject. Its publication played a large part in establishing that form of treatment on a solid foundation. Today, short-term psychotherapy is no longer viewed as a shabby stepsister to psychoanalysis and long-term psychoanalytic psychotherapy; Cinderella has at last come of age, decked out in the finery of widespread clinical usage and celebrated in a literature that now numbers hundreds of papers and monographs.

The basic principles and techniques of short-term anxiety-provoking psychotherapy (STAPP)—the particular form of brief therapy developed by Dr. Sifneos—remain much as they were presented in the earlier edition of this book. There have, however, been important developments over the past decade both in the field and in Dr. Sifneos's own conceptions. These have mandated a revised and expanded edition of the original volume in order to provide the reader with a review of the recent literature, a reassessment of the effectiveness of STAPP, a discussion of its expanded application to patients with somatic symptoms and abnormal grief reactions, and its usefulness in treating older persons.

A particular virtue of the earlier edition was its presentation of extensive verbatim material from the author's therapeutic sessions with his patients. That feature not only has been maintained in this volume but has been greatly expanded to include new clinical cases derived from Dr. Sifneos's continued practice and observation. Like its predecessor, this edition provides an excellent guide for the beginning psychiatrist and a reinvigorating inspiration for the seasoned therapist.

JOHN C. NEMIAH, M.D.

Foreword to the
First Edition

Short-term psychotherapy, although brief, is not ephemeral. In the decade or two of its existence, it has grown into a sturdy tree, and a sign of its maturity is the fact that it is now the subject of an increasing number of overview articles summarizing its literature and findings. Yet it remains a young and vigorous discipline. Its pioneers have not been elevated to a pantheon of venerable but mute immortals; on the contrary, they are to be found at the forefront of the field, actively contributing to the development of its theory and practice. This volume is ample testimony to their continued creativity.

Dr. Sifneos has lectured and written extensively about short-term anxiety-provoking psychotherapy (STAPP). Based on psychoanalytic principles, STAPP aims to resolve pathological psychic conflicts and help those suffering from them to learn new ways of being in their most intimate relationships. It does so by actively focusing the patients' sights on their Oedipal problems, and its effectiveness (given a proper selection of subjects by specific criteria) has been amply documented in controlled clinical studies.

One of the significant virtues of Dr. Sifneos's therapeutic techniques is that they can be systematically taught to the aspiring psychotherapist. Dr. Sifneos has touched briefly on his procedures here and there throughout his published writings, but detailed information about his approach has been restricted to those fortunate enough to have direct *viva voce* instruction through his didactic lectures and clinical supervision. Now, in this volume, he devotes his attention singly and entirely to the practical details of his method of short-term psychotherapy and does so with a clarity that arises from the demonstration of actual encounters with patients in therapeutic interviews. Step by step, Dr. Sifneos takes the reader through the evolution of the treatment process as this occurs with real individuals undergoing therapy.

The careful study of his exposition will not in itself make one an expert psychotherapist; that, of course, can come only from applying one's knowledge in the active, repeated practice of the art. But the reader can be assured of discovering exactly what he needs to know and do to become proficient in the therapeutic method Dr. Sifneos describes. That is the first and major step to effective and lasting learning.

JOHN C. NEMIAH, M.D.

Preface to the
Second Edition

During the past eight years the demand for short-term dynamic psychotherapy has continued to increase and, at the present time, this kind of treatment is offered to more and more patients, clearly establishing that it is a major addition to the therapist's armamentarium.

Criticism from those advocating the advantages of long-term psychotherapy, as well as the hostility of the news media, has diminished. Specificity has prevailed, and different types of psychotherapy of long-term or brief duration have been shown to be effective for well-selected groups of patients.

In the United States, despite the interest in short-term therapies shown by governmental agencies and third-party payers such as the insurance industries, no funds have been provided to support research on their outcome or the education of great numbers of mental health professionals who seek training in this field. As a result of this unfortunate state of affairs there exist very few centers in this country which offer the opportunity to develop the skills and learn the techniques of short-term dynamic psychotherapy.

It is significant, nevertheless, that the enthusiasm of a few workers in the field of short-term dynamic psychotherapy has remained high, and research studies using videotapes to demonstrate the evaluations, techniques, and outcome have helped to document the efficacy of their therapeutic modalities. In addition, many good books and articles have been published introducing new concepts, such as the importance of systematic case studies and personality styles by Horowitz, a variety of brief therapies by Budman, and an integrating model of time-limited psychotherapy by Strupp, to mention only a few.

The investigation of the efficacy of short-term anxiety-provoking psychotherapy (STAPP), which is the subject of this book, has continued during the last eight years, particularly in reference to patients with unresolved Oedipal conflicts. The chapter on outcome has therefore been expanded to include some of our findings.

Cautious attempts have also been made to utilize focal and innovating techniques for the treatment of individuals with borderline as well as compulsive personalities.

In this second edition an effort has been made to present the specific technical factors which seem to have a therapeutic effect, such as problem solving, self-understanding, and new learning, and which are utilized by the patients to solve new emotional conflicts long after the end of their treatment.

Chapters on the treatment of elderly patients and the handling of individuals with physical symptomatology have been added; a history of the extensive treatment of a male patient has been presented to complement the discussion of the therapy of my female patient which appears in Appendix I.

Finally, I want to express my gratitude to all those in practically every state in this country, as well as in Canada, Switzerland, Belgium, Holland, all of the Scandinavian countries, Italy, and Greece, who invited me to speak and who organized workshops where I could present my work and my videotapes. This invaluable support has been heartwarming and has become a motivating force for me to pursue this fascinating work. I am forever indebted to them.

PETER E. SIFNEOS

Preface to the
First Edition

During the last few years, dynamic psychotherapies of brief duration have suddenly become very popular. Although a few investigators studied these kinds of treatment methods systematically over a long period of time and were convinced of their effectiveness, the recent emphasis on primary care, the increased national health insurance coverage, and the documentation which has been provided pointing to tangible therapeutic results, even in patients with serious neurotic difficulties, have aroused a great deal of interest in these treatment modalities all over the world. The familiar criticisms from advocates of long-term psychotherapy are more subdued, and one hears less often the pompous pronouncement that psychotherapy is unscientific. For all intents and purposes, therefore, it seems that short-term psychotherapy is here to stay.

Time limitation is, of course, a crucial factor in all brief therapies, yet it is paradoxical that there is no consensus among the workers in this field as to exactly what is meant by this concept. It should be emphasized from the start, however, that the primary reason for shortening the time interval is not because of demands that more services be made available to patients in the community at large. Rather, the governing force behind any kind of therapeutic intervention should be the documentation that it is a treatment well suited to each patient's idiosyncratic needs. In this respect, certain kinds of brief therapy are indeed indicated for a fairly large group of well-selected patients.

Some of these issues have been dealt with in my book *Short-Term Psychotherapy and Emotional Crisis* (Sifneos, 1972) in a more general way. Because of a certain prevailing confusion, however, and to avoid misunderstandings, I shall elaborate my ideas about short-term dynamic psychotherapy more extensively in the present volume. Furthermore, instead of writing only one chapter about the evaluation of the patient and one on the technique, as I did in my previous book, I shall concentrate on presenting as systematically as possible the psychiatric evaluation of a well-selected group of patients. In addition, I shall give a detailed description of the technique of a specialized kind of psychotherapy of short duration, called "anxiety provoking." In order to illustrate convincingly what I am discussing, I have used as many verbatim clinical vignettes as possible so as not only to demonstrate as explicitly as I can how short-term dynamic psychotherapy should be performed but also to encourage many therapists to utilize it in their everyday practice.

"Anxiety-provoking" psychotherapy utilizes the patient's anxiety as a motivating force to help him resolve his difficulties. Because it is also of short-term duration, it will be referred from now on as STAPP (*Short Term Anxiety-Provoking Psychotherapy*).

STAPP is not the only kind of brief dynamic psychotherapy. Malan (1976a,b,c) has described a technique of brief psychotherapy which lasts up to 40 interviews. He has also demonstrated convincingly and brilliantly that he obtains successful results even with patients who have serious psychopathology and whom we would not have considered to be good candidates for STAPP. Mann (1973), with his 12-interview "time-limited psychotherapy," is able to deal successfully with individuals who have problems with separation and for whom his type of treatment is ideally suited.

Davanloo (1978) has ingeniously developed a broad-focused brief dynamic psychotherapy for individuals with incapacitating phobias and obsessive-compulsive symptomatology which, by creating a therapeutic alliance and then dealing head on with the defenses over a period of several months, is able to help them cope with the conflicts underlying their difficulties and to produce an impressive psychodynamic resolution of their problems.

There are others who offer modified forms of brief dynamic psychotherapy, such as Bellak and Small (1965), Barten (1971), McGuire (1965a,b, 1968; McGuire & Sifneos, 1970), Notman, Stracker, and many more in the United States and Canada. In Europe, Schneider (1976) and his group in Lausanne, Heiberg and her collaborators in Oslo, and Pierloot, Luminet, and Meyer in their respective departments in Louvain, Liège, and Hamburg have developed techniques with very promising results.

It seems obvious, therefore, that we are dealing with a variety of psychotherapeutic interventions of short-term duration all using psychodynamic principles, with some more indicated in a population of neurotic individuals with circumscribed difficulties, while others offer help to somewhat more seriously disturbed neurotic patients.

This book is about STAPP. This kind of treatment involves a dyadic interaction between the patient and the therapist which has affective, cognitive, and educational components. It is a focal, goal-oriented, psychodynamic psychotherapy which envisages that the patient is capable of cooperating with the therapist within the context of a therapeutic alliance, and is able to resolve the psychological conflicts underlying his difficulties. Thus the selection of appropriate candidates according to specified criteria is a *sine qua non*. The requirements for this treatment involve weekly, face-to-face interviews lasting 45 minutes. There is no specified number of interviews, nor is there a termination date set. Rather, the length of this therapy is tailor-made to fit each patient's time requirement to solve a specified problem which has been agreed upon between himself and his therapist. It may take 6, 9, 14, or at most 20 interviews. Although it is clearly understood between the two participants that the treatment will be brief, its termination is left open-ended.

The nature of the psychological conflicts which are chosen to be resolved, and which underlie the patient's difficulties, are Oedipal or triangular. This implies that problems must have developed between the patient and his parents during early childhood and are being repeated in his current interpersonal relations. These problems have to do with a competition with the parent of the same sex for the love and affection of the parent, or a parent surrogate, of the opposite sex. Repetitive unsuccessful attempts to deal with these conflicts give rise to circumscribed symptoms and/or to well-delineated interpersonal difficulties, which act as a compelling force in making the patient seek help.

The technical therapeutic considerations for this kind of psychotherapy are specific and clear-cut. The therapist must encourage the development of a therapeutic alliance and must create an atmosphere where learning can take place. Taking advantage of the prevailing positive transference feelings, staying within the specified focus, and using anxiety-provoking confrontation questions, clarifications, and interpretations, he must strive to avoid getting entangled in pregenital characterological issues, such as passivity, dependence, sadomasochistic or narcissistic features, and acting-out tendencies which are used defensively by the patient and which tend to prolong the treatment.

With attention to both the cognitive and the emotional components, new learning, self-understanding, and problem-solving techniques are systematically taught to the patient so as to bring about a "corrective emotional experience" and a dynamic resolution of the Oedipus complex. Finally, and as soon as evidence is provided in terms of tangible examples that changes are actually taking place, the therapy must come to an end.

This book, then, will present a detailed and factual account of STAPP. The first part describes the typical complaints presented by the patients and enumerates the steps that must be taken for the proper evaluation of their psychological difficulties. These include a systematic developmental history taking, a specification of selection criteria, and the establishment of a therapeutic contract.

The second part deals with a detailed discussion of the specific therapeutic techniques which are utilized, and which have already been outlined. Finally, the third part describes briefly the supervision of those who want to learn to offer this kind of therapy and the results which can be expected. As often as possible, clinical examples to enrich the theoretical discussion will be presented from interviews with patients who were seen over a 20-year period at the psychiatric clinics of the Massachusetts General and Beth Israel Hospitals of Harvard Medical School, and in my own private practice.

First and foremost, I want to express my gratitude to those patients who provided me with a rich clinical material without which this book would not have been possible. Careful attention has been paid in making all the necessary alterations to protect their confidentiality and to preserve their anonymity without distorting the relevance of the basic observations or the nature of the psychotherapeutic interactions.

To my close friend of many years, John Nemiah, I am deeply indebted for his cordial and continued encouragement in pursuing my work on STAPP in his department without any interference. It is a privilege for me to be a member of his department at Harvard, where an academic atmosphere predominates, where stimulating discussions take place, where novel ideas are developed, and where teaching and learning are possible. For all these things I want to express my appreciation to him.

Without the warm support, the careful reviewing, and the stimulating comments of my long-standing friend Freddy Frankel, this book would have been difficult to write. My special and grateful appreciation is deeply felt.

To George Fishman, for his meticulous attention to detail and for his stimulating discussion of my manuscript, I am grateful and indebted.

I am especially thankful to our short-term psychotherapy research team—Drs. Roberta Apfel, Ellen Bassuk, and Andrew Gill—for their constructive and critical discussions, both clinical and theoretical, and to Donald Fern, who was an active member of our team and whose loss is greatly felt.

The various therapists whom I had the privilege to supervise over many years, and who provided me with invaluable insights which I could utilize meaningfully in thinking about this therapy, have contributed greatly to my understanding of this treatment. I owe my thanks to them.

To my colleagues overseas—Drs. Habib Davanloo, Astrid Heiberg, Daniel Luminet, David Malan, Roland Pierloot, and Pierre Schneider and their assistants—I want to express my thanks for many thoughtful comments about short-term psychotherapy in general and my own work in particular.

Last but not least, however, to my secretaries, Beth Noonan and Phyllis Wiseman—gracious and patient—who deciphered my handwriting and on their own free time typed my manuscript, much credit is due. Their efforts are gratefully appreciated.

Finally, I want to express a feeling of prevailing helplessness when I try to recreate the lively atmosphere of the therapeutic interviews, or to recapture the warmth of the interaction with my patients. Adequate words cannot be found for the proper description of such a relationship. When the treatment comes to an end, however, the feelings of pride for a meaningful achievement and of sadness for the termination of a friendly relation usually give rise to an occasional tear which both patient and therapist want to hide, but which is evidence of the value and success of their brief human encounter.

PETER E. SIFNEOS

Boston, Massachusetts

Contents

PART TWO: TECHNIQUE

PART THREE: RESULTS

PART ONE

THE PSYCHIATRIC EVALUATION

CHAPTER 1

Certain Common Complaints of Prospective STAPP Patients

If one of the most important aspects of STAPP has to do with the selection of appropriate candidates according to criteria clearly specified during the psychiatric evaluation, it is important, first of all, to describe the kinds of problems which most of these patients complain about and which are often encountered among individuals in a psychiatric clinic population.

A detailed and qualitative study of the people who make up a psychiatric clinic population offers the opportunity to understand better the individuals who at times of stress develop psychological crises and who seek psychiatric help to overcome their difficulties.

Statistical data on age, sex, marital status, and occupation which are ordinarily used to describe a clinic population give only a superficial impression of the individual patients, while a very detailed case presentation, interesting though it may be, fails to characterize the whole group.

It should be emphasized that a psychiatric clinic population is not usually balanced in terms of race, ethnic group, age, sex, and education. Rather, it is composed of individuals who despite their efforts to overcome their problems have failed, and who have decided on their own, or following the advice of someone else, to seek psychiatric assistance (Sifneos, 1972).

Patients should not be selected, however, on the basis of their expressed needs or demands. The unfortunate tendency toward consumerism, when the patient is viewed as someone who can go shopping and select the product of his choice, is silly and dangerous. The heroin addict threatens to harm others in order to get heroin; the anxious borderline character demands tranquilizing medication for immediate alleviation of the discomfort which he experiences. Despite these expressed demands, however, we should not give heroin to the addict, nor chlorpromazine to the borderline character, since eliminating the anxiety will merely perpetuate its raison d'être. Similarly, we should not offer psychotherapy, even if the patient asks for it, when in our professional opinion it is contraindicated—and many times it is.

How, then, does one go about evaluating the psychological difficulties presented to us by patients so as to help them get the expert help which they need? The first step is to survey the kinds of complaints which patients verbalize and which are instrumental in motivating them to seek psychiatric help.

For STAPP candidates, the commonly encountered problems are usually certain circumscribed symptoms, such as anxiety, phobias, depressions, and mild obsessive-compulsive symptoms of sudden onset, as well as a variety of interpersonal difficulties.

ANXIETY

Anxiety alone is one of the most common complaints we encounter. Here is an example:

A 30-year-old housewife described the onset of acute anxiety in the parking lot of a shopping center which necessitated her immediate return to her home. From then on, she asked her neighbor and friend to accompany her during her shopping expeditions.

She described these anxiety attacks as "absurd happenings" because she realized that they were not associated with any realistic frightening events. She also emphasized her annoyance with her helplessness and her inability to control her anxiety. When she was asked to describe this feeling of helplessness, she went on as follows: "Well, I don't want to give you the wrong impression. I exaggerated a minute ago. What I really meant to say was that it was more comfortable to have Claire accompany me. I felt convinced, however, that if I had to, I could endure this anxiety, and that if I was forced to, I could do my own shopping. It was easier, however, to have my friend with me."

When she was asked to describe the events surrounding the onset of her symptom, she claimed at first that there was nothing specific to which she could attribute them. The following exchange took place with the clinic evaluator:

PATIENT: Last week I had a doctor's appointment because for the last few weeks I have had some burning on urination, and on one occasion I observed a little bit of blood in my urine. I was worried about it and I talked to my husband, who suggested that I should consult Dr. R. I made an appointment. He was very nice and reassuring, but he suggested that I should see a urologist and he gave me the name of a specialist. Two days before this anxiety attack I went to see the new doctor. I remember noticing his car with the M.D. plates parked right in front of his office because it was a Buick, and because it reminded me of my father, who always drives a Buick. During the examination, I was quite apprehensive but I had no anxiety attack, nothing like what happened later on. I remember that it was somewhat painful, and I was worried that the doctor might find something wrong. He was also very nice and made it as pleasurable as he possibly could, which reminded me of the time when I was eleven years old when I fell from my bike and bruised my thigh. I remember crying, but my father sat me on his lap, examined the cut, and said that it was going to be all right.

EVALUATOR: Why did this bike episode come to your mind right now?

PATIENT: First of all, I remember being reassured by my dad, and then it was this car—the Buick—as I told you already.

EVALUATOR: Go on.

PATIENT: Well, come to think of it . . . it is strange, but I just remembered that when I went shopping at the center, when I got my anxiety attack, I had parked my car next to another Buick. The funny thing is that at that moment—I had completely forgotten this until now—I felt suddenly anxious and the notion of driving back and asking Claire to accompany me crossed my mind.

It was clear by the end of the evaluation that this patient's anxiety was related to her urological examination and the pleasure which she received after the doctor's reassurances, which was also associated to the earlier episode with her father, to whom she was very much attached.

ANXIETY IN CONJUNCTION WITH OTHER SYMPTOMS

Anxiety may also be associated with a variety of physical symptoms. Here is an example of anxiety and hyperventilation:

A 20-year-old male college student complained of a sudden onset of panicky feelings, excessive perspiration, and hyperventilation. Although these symptoms had occurred off and on in a very mild form for seven years, the suddenness and intensity of their onset seemed to have taken the patient by surprise. The course of events was as follows: The patient had attended a football game. His college team had won, and he was feeling quite happy. On his way out he met some friends who invited him to a postgame party. He had quite a lot to drink and noticed that he had a vague feeling of uneasiness whenever he thought of returning to his dorm. When two of his friends suggested a tour of the local bars, he welcomed the opportunity to go along with them. At one of the bars, two prostitutes approached them, and the patient, although surprised by his behavior—he had never before gone out with a prostitute—immediately accepted the invitation to go with one of them. He found himself impotent, however, although he had never before had such difficulty and had had considerable sexual experience in the past with a variety of women. The prostitute ridiculed him and asked him to pay her twice the amount of money that she usually charged because the experience was so unpleasant to her and had wounded her pride. The patient felt humiliated, paid what she had asked without objecting, and left. He went back to his dorm and slept for twelve hours. He remembered that he had a series of unpleasant dreams but could not recall their content. He woke up in a cold sweat and started to hyperventilate. He could not get rid of an irrelevant thought which had to do with the prostitute's wearing a blond wig which she took off when they entered her hotel room. He noticed that her hair was actually dark and that she looked much older than he had expected: "She was in her late thirties instead of her early twenties as I had originally thought." He remembered that the phrase "with an older woman" went through his head while he was impotent and had also popped into his mind just before he started to hyperventilate.

The patient was an only son and was very much attached to his parents. His mother had died when he was 15 years old, and he remembered being very upset and crying during her funeral. The mild anxiety attacks, which he had mentioned, increased in frequency after his mother's death but subsided after a while.

PHOBIA WITH OBSESSIVE THOUGHTS

Phobias are the second most common symptom which we have encountered. Here is an example:

A 17-year-old high school student became afraid of contracting a venereal disease following his first sexual experience with an older girl whom he met at a party. He described how, at first, following the sexual intercourse, he felt happy and satisfied with the thought that he was "a real man." When he subsequently called the girl and asked her for a date, she refused, claiming that she had a steady boyfriend. He was very upset by this rejection and tried to convince her to change her mind, but he was unsuccessful. Following the telephone call he started to have doubts about his sexual performance. He went on as follows:

PATIENT: I started to think that maybe she didn't like me, or that I had not satisfied her, although at the time she had given me the impression that she liked it. Then I started to think that my penis was too small and that I couldn't make her have an orgasm. The idea then occurred to me that maybe she had intercourse with some other guys in the same way she did with me. Suddenly the thought that she may have a venereal disease popped into my head. I felt a cold sinking sensation in my stomach. I thought that she got it from her boyfriend or some other guy.

From then on I couldn't stop thinking about V.D. I felt depressed and I started to read everything I could lay my hands on that described venereal diseases. The more I read, the more I became preoccupied and the more my fear increased. I started to get panicky.

I borrowed a dermatology book which belonged to a friend of my older brother, who was a medical student. I read about the symptoms of gonorrhea. I felt pretty good after that because I didn't have any burning on urination or any discharge, but when I read about syphilis, and how it appears in three to four weeks, I again broke into a cold sweat. "Oh, my God," I thought, "how can I wait three or four weeks? It would be real torture." From then on the only thought I had was about V.D. I couldn't bear it any longer, so I spoke to my brother Joe, who made an appointment for me to see a doctor. I felt relieved for a while after the doctor examined me and reassured me that I was okay, but this feeling didn't last for long. Thoughts and doubts about the doctor started creeping in. With all the reading I had done, I had become an expert on venereal diseases. I thought, "Why didn't the doctor give me a Hinton test? He said I didn't have syphilis. How did he know? Maybe I have another type of illness." All these thoughts kept going around in my head, and made me miserable. Finally, I decided that I should talk to my mother and tell her everything.

His mother listened carefully and was very reassuring but suggested to the patient that it would be advantageous to him to talk to his father, since he was more experienced in "all these things." The patient felt very frightened by this suggestion and begged his mother not to mention anything to his father. "Dad would never understand," he said. Later on, when he thought about it a little longer, he decided that it was a good idea after all, but that it was up to him to talk to his father. He talked with his father, who suggested psychotherapy to him. It was following this that the patient went to see a psychiatrist.

GRIEF REACTION

Three months after the sudden death of his wife, a 42-year-old father of two children became depressed, slept poorly, ate infrequently, and had difficulty in concentrating on his work because he kept thinking about his dead wife and experiencing feelings of guilt. What seemed to have precipitated his depression was the unusual attention paid to him by his neighbor, a 48-year-old widow who had suggested that they live together. Although he loved his wife and had described his marriage as a happy one, he did not seem to have experienced feelings of sadness after her death. His neighbor friend was very helpful to him during that period. She made all the funeral arrangements and was very supportive of the patient's two teenage sons.

The patient was always very close to his two elderly parents, who were described as strict and very religious, and who lived close by. They were also very fond of his deceased wife and disapproved of the attention paid to him by his widow friend. On one occasion, his mother had spoken very critically of his neighbor. "It was like giving me a lecture, a mother talking to a child, not a grown-up man." He also added that his mother said that there was no comparison between his wife and his friend, and suggested that he "remarry a younger woman." This took the patient by surprise because, although he admitted that he liked his neighbor, enjoyed her company, and appreciated her help, the thought of marrying her had not crossed his mind, and he resented his mother's implication. When his friend suggested moving in with him, he was "thunderstruck" but soon the idea appealed to him. It was following this realization that he started feeling apprehensive. He kept thinking more and more about his dead wife and had strong feelings of guilt whenever the thought of his widow friend crossed his mind. It was at the suggestion of his friend that he called the clinic for an appointment.

When he was seen it was clear that the patient had already started to grieve over his wife's death, although this had been somewhat delayed. It was thought that he required only a few interviews to straighten out his feelings for his mother, his dead wife, and his neighbor, and to overcome his guilt.

MILD DEPRESSION

A 30-year-old lawyer complained of feeling depressed every time he had satisfactory sexual intercourse with his wife. During these times, he tended to blame himself for not spending more time on his legal work and for being interested in sex instead. He said that he had lived with his wife for two years before they were married and had had no sexual difficulties or guilt feelings, but he described sexual intercourse as relatively unsatisfactory. It was after they were married, however, that he experienced depressive feelings for the first time after a sexual encounter with his wife which they both had particularly enjoyed—when she announced that she had had an orgasm for the first time in her life.

The patient had lost his parents in a plane accident when he was nine years old and was brought up by his maternal grandmother. His grandfather, whom he adored, died of a heart attack when the patient was 16, and he indicated that he felt very bad for a long time afterward. His grades slipped in high school, and he broke off his relationship with his steady girlfriend quite impulsively, without being able to understand his real motivation for this act.

Following her husband's death, his grandmother became very attached to the patient and depended on him for financial advice and in other matters. She also became jealous of his girlfriend. When asked if this jealousy had something to do with breaking off his relation with his girlfriend, he said that he had never given it thought before, but he considered it possible. From then on, he remembered becoming apprehensive whenever he became interested in women, particularly sexually. This state of affairs became progressively worse, and he started to feel very stifled by his grandmother's dependence on him. When he left for college, he felt relieved but also experienced guilt feelings. While in law school he met his future wife, whom he described as "prudish," which he felt was not true because it was she who suggested that they live together, and it was he who wanted to get married.

As mentioned already, their sexual relations were uneventful before their marriage, but not particularly satisfying. After his wife had an orgasm, he became depressed and remained so until he finally decided to seek psychiatric help.

In a subsequent chapter, I shall emphasize that the issues on which the therapist attempts to focus during the psychiatric evaluation of STAPP patients, and on which he concentrates his attention during the therapy, must be Oedipal problems. In these last two case examples, the patients had experienced major losses which, it may be argued, could easily have become the therapeutic focus of their brief therapy. This has not been the case, however. After a thorough evaluation of these patients, it was clear that unresolved Oedipal issues were the problem to be dealt with during their psychotherapy. It was also clear that the first patient had already resolved his grief about his wife's death, whereas the difficulties and guilt feelings about his neighbor had to be straightened out. In the second patient, it was obvious that his grandmother had become a parental substitute and that she was also endowed with unresolved sexual feelings which had been displaced on the patient's wife.

INTERPERSONAL DIFFICULTIES

Of all the problems which motivated patients to seek help because of their wishes to change, the commonest complaints we encountered involved interpersonal difficulties. Here is an example:

A 25-year-old female single graduate student complained of disappointment and irritation at herself for repeated failures in her relationships with men. She described her feelings as follows:

PATIENT: I have had problems with men ever since I can remember. What I find most annoying is that I like men, and when I meet someone, at first I get along very well with him. I know that I'm attractive and that men like me. When I meet a fellow that I feel attracted to at a party, I flirt with him and I enjoy the experience very much. A few dates later I know that I'll end up in bed with him. This happens, and it's usually quite enjoyable, and then—and this is what disturbs me—I start giving double messages. I don't know why I do it, but at least now I recognize that I do, while a few years ago I didn't. (*When asked to give an example, she went on*): When I was discussing Vietnam with Joe—my last boyfriend—I agreed with what he was saying, yet I could hear myself starting to object to some of his remarks when I knew that he was perfectly right. It was as if something powerful had come out of me that said, "Janet, argue even if you agree." I know this is perfectly silly. Well, what happened was that Joe and I ended up having a fight. When we tried to have sex, it wasn't as good as it had been before. From then on, things started to deteriorate.

There were more and more meaningless arguments and less and less good sex. Joe asked me why I behaved the way I did. It was really pathetic. I knew he was right. I know he was trying desperately and for the last time to save our relationship, but you know what came out of me at that time? Well, it wasn't very nice. I said, "Joe, you're a bigot, you're to blame for ruining a good relationship. It's all your fault." I knew all along that it wasn't true, yet I enjoyed saying it. Making a long story short, we decided to end it all. What is so sad is that I liked Joe, and this attitude has become a habit with me. The same thing happened with Paul, and with Les. Of course, I always feel bad afterward, but I have the idea that the whole thing is predetermined, that there's nothing I can do to stop it, and that my relations with men are always doomed to fail. Of course I know this is all nonsense, and this is why I am here.

The patient was aware that her difficulties had started when her brother was born. She was five years old at that time and she had been her parents' favorite. She knew that her older sister was jealous of her. After her brother's birth, however, her parents started showing evidence of favoritism for him. She denied any jealous feelings, however, and remembered that she had the fantasy that he was a doll who belonged to her. During her early adolescence she was prematurely interested in boys and remembered her mother's remarking to her father that "Janet will get married very young." This infuriated the patient, but she was pleased to hear her father answer, "No, I don't think so. She is too much attached to her brother." The patient felt that there was truth in this remark and she thought that her relation with her father and brother was the key to her difficulties with men.

These case examples are fairly typical of what one hears from prospective STAPP candidates. It is not my intention at this point, however, to describe the psychodynamics of these patients' problems. This will be discussed in the following chapters.

Here is another example:

A 30-year-old female college student came to the clinic complaining of difficulties of six months' duration in her relations with her boyfriend. She also added that her mother had been seriously ill and there was a possibility that she was suffering from cancer. She said that as a child she did not have a good relationship with her mother, but that recently they had become closer together. The following exchange then took place between the evaluator and the patient:

EVALUATOR: Now which of the two problems is responsible for your coming here to the psychiatric clinic? Your mother's illness or your difficulties with your boyfriend?
PATIENT: I have had a lot of time to think about my mother's illness. It is very sad, but I am prepared for any eventuality; on the other hand, I cannot understand what is happening in my relationship with my boyfriend.
EVALUATOR: Now then, what exactly is the problem?
PATIENT: Ever since October I have been feeling irritable with Joe. He annoys me, yet there is nothing which happened to account for this feeling in me. I think that I have changed in reference to him and it is unfair because he has remained the same. He has done nothing to contribute to or to cause this dissatisfaction in me.
EVALUATOR: Are you sure that nothing has happened?
PATIENT: Not at face value, but in September our friendship has changed, our relationships became sexual, but in the past this has happened with other men.
EVALUATOR: You mean that a friendship which has turned into a sexual relationships has become a problem?
PATIENT: Yes, two or three times, but it was different with these other men. The sexual relationships was completely unsatisfactory, while with Joe it is very satisfactory. Furthermore, I like Joe much more than these other men . . . (looking pensive)
EVALUATOR: Go on please.
PATIENT: There is something else, however, which is also special. You see, Joe is six years older than I am.
EVALUATOR: In what way is this of significance?
PATIENT: You see, all the men I have been dating up to now have been younger.
EVALUATOR: Why did you date younger men?
PATIENT: It is safe. Younger men are immature and they are easy to deal with. I don't become attached to them. I am protecting myself.

EVALUATOR: Why do you want to protect yourself? What comes to your mind?

PATIENT: My older brother. He always wanted to be protective and he did protect me. I was very close to him, particularly after my father died when I was thirteen. Then he left to go to college and I did not see him for years because after college he was in the marines in Vietnam. I missed him. I became upset when he left.

EVALUATOR: Did you have the same feeling of wanting to be protected and actually being protected by Joe?

PATIENT: In a funny sort of a way I did.

EVALUATOR: Why do you say "funny"?

PATIENT: You see, I hadn't thought of it in that way, but both my brother and Joe are six years older than I am.

EVALUATOR: So there is a connection between the two. Now when you were young was there any sex play with your brother?

PATIENT (blushing): Yes, there was. My brother used to come to my room and fondle me, but I always pretended that I was asleep. When I grew older I started feeling guilty. I became irritable.

EVALUATOR: So is this the reason why you are irritable with Joe, because you feel guilty about having sexual relations with someone who reminds you of your brother?

PATIENT: I never thought of it, but on second thought it seems quite obvious.

It may be significant to point out that even in the early part of the evaluation interview, important connections can be made between feelings which the patients have had for people in the past and those for individuals with whom the patients are currently involved.

These two examples are fairly typical of the types of interpersonal difficulties which brought patients to the psychiatric clinic seeking help in disentangling these relationships.

For all intents and purposes, using DSM-III criteria, most of these patients could be diagnosed as "adjustment disorders" or adjustment disorders with anxious or depressed mood.

CHAPTER 2

History Taking and Reformulation of the Presenting Complaints

---

Having obtained all the information he can about the patient's presenting complaints, how does the evaluator go about deciding whether or not the patient is someone who would benefit from STAPP? In this and the next two chapters I shall describe the steps that are necessary to accomplish this task. There are four integral factors which are involved in the overall evaluation process:

1. The complete biographical history taking and reformulation of the presenting complaints
2. The specific criteria for selection for STAPP
3. The psychodynamic formulation, therapeutic focus, and contract
4. The specification of criteria for successful outcome

A word of caution should be added at this point so as not to give the impression that each one of these four factors is a separate entity or that it is independent of the others. Rather, it is crucial that the evaluation process be understood as a global assessment of the patient's psychopathology which the evaluator must scrutinize extensively. Although the evaluator should try to formulate appropriately these four parameters, they are presented here simply as helpful guidelines to be followed by the evaluator during the patient's initial work-up.

At the outset, the emphasis should always be on the evaluator. Despite the fact that it is the patient who possesses all the necessary information which, if sorted out appropriately, will throw light on the nature of his psychological problem, he does not have the expertness or the objectivity to give it the proper perspective. Thus he must rely on the evaluator's professional knowledge and skill to help him formulate it correctly.

Obviously, this evaluation should become a joint problem-solving venture, involving two people who have distinctive goal-directed tasks. It is important, therefore, that during the evaluation process there should always be a "psychological division of labor."

HISTORY TAKING

Obtaining a good history is probably the single most important aspect of the psychological evaluation. The way the evaluator guides the patient to provide him with a historical account of his life can become the basis of understanding the nature of the patient's difficulties as well as of solving them. There are several principles about history taking which must be adhered to.

1. It should take place sometime during the middle of the first interview, after the patient has had an opportunity to describe his presenting complaints.

2. The evaluator should ask the patient to recall the earliest memory or event in his life, even if this is an episode which he has only heard about from his parents or relatives at a later time. The recollection of the earliest memory usually throws some light on the way in which the patient subsequently views his life. Individuals who tend to remember some terrible event do, in some way, emphasize that the view of their life is an unhappy one. On the contrary, a happy event or a pleasant memory from the patient communicates a sense of ease about life which is significant in pointing out that the problems to be encountered are not likely to be very serious.

3. Specific information should be obtained about the structure of the patient's family and the atmosphere which prevailed while he was growing up. Here are two examples:

A young female student came to the clinic at the insistence of her mother, who was worried about her repeated bouts of overeating and subsequent weight gain. When she was asked to talk about her first and earliest memory, the patient insisted that she did not remember anything before the age of nine years. The evaluator tried for a while to prod her into remembering events earlier than that time, but he was unsuccessful. After completing the history taking, which pointed to severe defects in her character, poor relations with people, intensely ambivalent feelings for her mother, and periods of bulimia (abnormal cravings for food), the evaluator learned that on several occasions during her life these episodes were followed by bouts of starvation dieting and severe weight loss. Once more he inquired about her earliest memory. She was silent for a while and then, looking very apprehensive, mentioned that she remembered her mother's telling her that when she was four years old, her father had been drafted into the army during World War II. Her mother took her to the airport to see her father depart, but she seemed to have become terrified by the noise of the airplane propellers. She screamed and screamed, so much so that she turned "blue" because she could not breathe. The patient went on as follows: "I guess that episode shows you how unhappy I was way back then—I have always been very unhappy. I think that I didn't want to tell you this story when you first asked me because it was so sad. It points to the fact that, from the very earliest part of my life, I was terrified. I was scared. I was in a panic. I have been feeling this way ever since." When the evaluator asked her why she volunteered to tell him about this early episode after the history taking was almost over, she was quiet for a while and then said, "At first you didn't know anything about me. I wanted to give you a good impression, but, after I told you all my problems, I guess it didn't make any difference anyway." She looked very depressed and burst into tears.

It was obvious that this young woman was seriously ill. It was clear that she needed long-term supportive psychotherapy.

On the contrary, a 24-year-old electronics technician became ecstatic when he recalled his earliest memory as follows:

PATIENT: I must have been four or five. In any case I was in my room sitting on the floor and playing with my cars. I was happy and peaceful. I remember that my mother came into my room.

She announced that dinner was ready, but I asked her to sit down and wait for a few minutes so I could finish putting all my cars back in their garage. She smiled and sat down by the window. I looked up and there was my beautiful mother! The sun was exactly behind her, so I couldn't see her face, but her long blond hair was sparkling. It looked like a shining golden crown. I walked up to her and told her that she looked like the fairy queen in my coloring book. She put her arms around me and gave me a kiss. I never forgot how happy I felt at that moment!

It is possible that the patient felt a little too happy because this attachment to his mother and his unsuccessful search for a substitute created some problems later on in his life in his relations with women. In any case, these problems were dealt with appropriately during his STAPP, from which he obtained much benefit.

4. The nature of the relationship with each parent is, of course, vital and must be scrutinized, because it always throws light on two of the selection criteria for STAPP (described in detail in the next chapter). Thus, first of all, one must investigate and get a perspective on what kinds of parents the patient had and what they actually did for the patient. Their ability to provide security or safety to their growing child, for example, should be kept in mind as well as their ability to teach him to anticipate trouble, to postpone instant gratification, and to tolerate anxiety and displeasure. All these help the child feel secure and provide him with a solid background which helps him develop and mature. Emphasis should then be placed on the specific interactions that have taken place between the patient—as an individuated, separate human being—and each one of his parents. As will be discussed subsequently, this assessment is important because it helps throw light on the Oedipal period and the problems which appeared during that time, and will become the therapeutic focus for this kind of short-term treatment.

Here are a few of the types of questions which should be asked in reference to the patient's interaction with his parents: What was your mother like? What was her personality like? What did she look like? What did she do for you? What did you do for her? What did you do together? Were you your mother's favorite? Was someone else her favorite? Did you prefer your mother to your father? How did your parents get along together? Did your relationship with your mother change? If so, at what time did it change? What was this relationship like when you were four years old? When you were seven? Was it the same? What about puberty and late adolescence? What is it like now? How can you summarize your relationship with your mother?

Similar questions should be asked in reference to the patient's father. In addition, detailed information should be obtained about the relations with each brother or sister, and with other key members of the family.

The patient should not be permitted to globalize in an effort to generalize and avoid anxiety. He should always be asked to give specific examples of events, episodes, memories, or fantasies which he may have had in reference to these vital relationships. For example, when the patient tends to answer vaguely a specific question about his father or mother, he is trying to avoid it. Usually one of the two most common ways which are used to bypass such an inquiry has to do with a patient's tendency to refer to his "parents" rather than to each parent separately. In that case, the evaluator should repeat his question and emphasize that he wants information specifically about each parent separately. He is convinced that, by globalizing, the patient is trying to run away from feelings which have been aroused as a result of his questions.

5. Following the assessment of the key relationships in the family, the evaluator should proceed to gather data about the patient's move from home to school, get a picture of his relations with teachers and peers, as well as obtain information about his academic performance or problems which might have appeared during that time.

6. Puberty is another period which will help throw light on the patient's successful or unsuccessful strivings to resolve the Oedipal transactions. Here are some questions which could be asked: How old were you when you started to menstruate? Were you prepared? How did your mother react to it? Did she help you? What were your feelings in reference to it? Were you frightened or did you feel proud at becoming a young woman? Did your father's feelings for you change? What about your brothers' or your sisters' feelings? Did your feelings for each of them change? If so, in what way? How did your friends react to it? Similar questions, of course, should be asked of male patients about their own experiences during puberty.

7. Questions about adolescence, with special emphasis on interpersonal relations at high school or college, should follow the data gathering on puberty; again, the evaluator should inquire about the patient's academic performance.

8. In addition, information about early adulthood will bring the evaluator an assessment of the patient's current life in terms of work, intellectual achievements, and interpersonal relations, as well as critical life events such as marriage, separations, and divorce.

9. Finally, a good medical history, including a system review, a sexual history, and a formal mental status evaluation, should complete the history taking.

Throughout all this time the evaluator must pay attention to the patient's appearance, style of relating, emotional reactions, posture, facial expressions, language and vocabulary, or any other verbal or nonverbal cues.

What I have tried to emphasize here is the attention which the evaluator must pay to obtain a thorough history. I offer a sample of the kinds of questions which should be asked. These are far from being exhaustive, however, and the evaluator should remember to look for and investigate the specific problems which are presented to him in each and every case.

Before going further, a word should be said about the nature of the type of questioning which is utilized by the evaluator. There are two kinds of questions which are ordinarily used: "open-ended questions," to which the patient responds by talking freely, and "forced-choice questions," in which the patient is expected to answer with a yes or a no. It is obvious that the exclusive use of one kind of questioning at the expense of the other invariably gives poor results. Judicious utilization of both types depends on the evaluator's skill and his wish to obtain information as complete as possible.

REFORMULATION OF THE PATIENT'S PRESENTING COMPLAINTS

So far the evaluator has heard about the patient's presenting complaints and has obtained a systematic history of his psychological development on a longitudinal basis. Now the evaluator's task is to synthesize this information into a psychodynamic hypothesis which will help explain the nature of the patient's psychological problem and set the stage for its resolution. Therefore, it is important that the evaluator attempt to recast the presenting complaints into a psychodynamic setting which will be acceptable to the patient. Some patients are almost able to do this by themselves and require very little assistance from the evaluator. Here is an example:

A 25-year-old graduate student had presented her problem at the beginning of the evaluation interview as follows: "I am anxious in my relations with my boyfriends because I tend to put on an act and pretend that I am someone that I am not. It is like wearing a mask. I want to free myself from this pattern of behavior."

After a systematic history had been obtained, with little assistance from the evaluator, the patient was able to present what she wanted to achieve as a result of her psychotherapy in the following way: "What has become very clear to me as a result of our discussion is that this behavior pattern of mine, which I dislike so much and which I want to get rid of, has its origin at the time when I was young and when I was trying to impress my father that I knew more than I really did. He would always see through my act and used to laugh and laugh whenever I tried it; yet, I kept trying over and over to impress him. His laughter was his rejection of me. The same thing happened with my last boyfriend, Larry."

This patient was able, as a result of one interview, to trace the origin of her behavior pattern with adult males to her relationship with her father during her childhood. The therapeutic focus is actually set by the patient in this case, and it is in agreement with the evaluator's psychodynamic formulation.

Other patients, on the other hand, require more assistance from their evaluators. Here is an example:

After the end of her history taking, a 30-year-old female housewife who worked part time at an insurance office was somewhat unsure as to which of the several problems that had brought her to the clinic bothered her most. These included her anger at her mother, her difficulties with other female employees at work, and her problems with her husband. When asked by the evaluator to assign priority only to one of these difficulties, she went on as follows:

PATIENT: All three problems seem to be equally important to me.

EVALUATOR: I understand, but let's look at it this way. Now, what was it that prompted you to call the clinic to set up this appointment?

PATIENT: The fight that I had with my mother on the telephone.

EVALUATOR: So maybe this is the most important problem.

PATIENT: No, because as I mentioned before, I had a fight with one of the girls at work which preceded my fight with my mother. She yelled at me for no apparent reason, and I kept thinking about it all day. When I talked to Bill, my husband, he was sympathetic, but I knew that he was busy. He has a lot of work to do for his bar exam. I was tense and I wanted to talk to someone. In any case, Bill isn't a good listener. He doesn't like people who complain, and that's another problem.

EVALUATOR: Is this then the problem?

PATIENT: Oh, no. I did think I needed some help, so I thought of calling my mother and asking her advice.

EVALUATOR: So?

PATIENT: Well, I did, and guess what my mother said? She said it was all my fault. She didn't even let me finish my story. She said, "Fay, you always become the victim and you always have a tendency to blame others." She said I used to do the same thing when I was a little girl. She went on and on, so I said, "Thanks, mother, for being such a help," and I hung up. I was mad. I kept thinking about my conversation with my mother and I couldn't sleep that night.

EVALUATOR: So the question is whether you were more angry at the girl at the office or at your mother after that telephone call.

PATIENT: It's interesting the way you put it. I hadn't thought of connecting the two episodes. I had looked at them separately. Actually, the girl at the office was criticizing me for being a victim in the same way my mother did. So the anger at both of them was the same.

EVALUATOR: So what is it that you want to accomplish out of all these things?

PATIENT: I want to get rid of everything.

EVALUATOR: You must choose only one. Which one will it be?

PATIENT: You aren't very helpful.

EVALUATOR: I really am. You see, helping you decide to place prior-

ity on your most important problem is giving you the right perspective on your difficulties, and you keep the decision in your
own hands.

PATIENT: I see what you mean . . . well, the anger at my mother, I
think, is the key to all the other problems. It's been simmering for
a long time. I suppose that it's my main difficulty, and I want to
understand it.

Although the patient had been unable at first to circumscribe
her difficulties, as a result of the history taking and the encouragement of the evaluator, who gently kept prodding her, by the end of
the evaluation interview she was ready to come to her own decision
about the problem she wanted to resolve.

The final point which should be mentioned in reference to the
history taking and reformulation of the patient's presenting complaints has to do with the evaluator's knowledge of the criteria for
selection of STAPP, which he must keep in mind as he collects information from the patient.

These criteria for selection will be discussed in detail in the
next chapter.

CHAPTER 3

Criteria for Selection for STAPP

A prerequisite for any kind of psychotherapy of short duration has to do with the discovery of the various common personality characteristics which are shared by those patients who are good candidates to receive it. Thus the specification of selection criteria for appropriate candidates becomes one of the first tasks of the psychiatric evaluation.

At present we have formulated very clearly our criteria for selection for STAPP, but this has taken a long time and it has not been easy. In my book *Short-Term Psychotherapy and Emotional Crisis* (Sifneos, 1972), I described how we treated our first STAPP patient and how he became the prototype for the development of selection criteria for this type of treatment. The original criteria which were used at the psychiatric clinic of the Massachusetts General Hospital for selecting STAPP patients were so strict that over a period of four years we were able to find only 50 appropriate candidates (Sifneos, 1961).

The findings on 21 out of the 50 patients who were seen in follow-up, over a period of six months to two years, were presented to Dr. Franz Alexander, who discussed my paper at the meetings of the American Psychiatric Association in 1960. He suggested that we liberalize our criteria for selection so as to help find a greater number of patients who would be considered as eligible candidates to receive STAPP. Stimulated by his comments, as well as receiving invaluable encouragement to continue this work from Dr. Elizabeth Zetzel, I was able to modify our selection criteria. This was achieved by dropping the criterion requiring the patient to be in a state of crisis. Patients in crisis usually visited the emergency floor of a hospital and were seen by whoever was assigned to work there. The staff, therefore, differed from those who worked in the psychiatric clinic and were evaluating patients for STAPP. Because of this administrative setup we had been unable to see psychiatric patients in crisis at the clinic. By eliminating the need for the patient to be in crisis as a criterion for selection, we started to look for patients who had developed circumscribed psychological difficulties over a certain period of time. Furthermore, it became clear that patients in a state of psychological crisis required a different kind of intervention, which has as its aim the provision of immediate assistance to the patient so as to overcome the crisis and help him to return to the state of emotional equilibrium which existed before the onset of the crisis.

As a result, two different kinds of psychotherapy dealing with crisis have been developed (described elsewhere; Sifneos, 1967). These are *crisis support* and *crisis intervention*. By modifying our selection criteria for STAPP, on the other hand, we were able during the next four years to test over 500 patients and to study the outcome of their treatment systematically.

During the Sixth International Congress of Psychotherapy held in London in 1964, the findings on these patients (Sifneos, 1965) were presented to a large number of participants as well as to Professors Sir Aubrey Lewis and Erich Lindemann. During the discussion, it became clear that a controlled study of outcome was necessary so as to validate as well as possible the general observations regarding the efficacy of STAPP. Such a research project was developed and its results are described in *The Role of Learning in Psychotherapy* (Porter, 1968).

Another unexpected and pleasurable event took place in London in 1964. It involved the accidental meeting with Dr. David Malan and the discovery that he was conducting similar work at the Tavistock Clinic, and that similar observations about selection criteria, techniques, and outcome were being made on patients receiving short-term dynamic psychotherapy.

Over the ensuing years our work on criteria for selection was continued and perfected. The following criteria for selection are those which we use at the present time:

1. The ability of the patient to have a circumscribed chief complaint
2. Evidence of a give and take, or "meaningful relationship" with another person during early childhood
3. Capacity to relate flexibly to the evaluator during the interview and to experience and express feelings freely
4. Psychological sophistication—above average intelligence and psychological mindedness
5. Motivation for change and not for symptom relief

CIRCUMSCRIBED CHIEF COMPLAINT

In the previous chapters I gave examples of the types of complaints which STAPP patients usually present, and how it is the responsibility of the evaluator to help the patient reformulate his complaints, following the history taking, so as to simplify their joint therapeutic task.

The ability to circumscribe denotes a capacity to choose one out of a variety of problems which the patient considers to be of importance and to assign to it top priority for resolution. The ability to make such a choice is an indication that the patient has considerable capabilities, that he can tolerate a certain degree of anxiety, and that he has the potential to withstand stress. All these assets of character point to the presence of strengths which can be utilized effectively during the short-term treatment, a treatment which is focal and which constantly necessitates making choices and reaching decisions.

Looked at from a different point of view, assigning top priority to the one problem which must be solved during the treatment denotes the effective use of isolation by the patient. This defense mechanism, which helps phobic patients create a symptom and enables them to deal with the anxiety resulting from their underlying psychological conflicts, has the effect of diffusing the anxiety by making it more tolerable.

The ability to circumscribe points further to the patient's capability to select a whole area of conflicting wishes rather than simply to choose a superficial symptom or interpersonal difficulty. Such a capacity, of course, demonstrates that the awareness of the underlying conflicts whose resolution will enable him to eliminate his symptoms once and for all is present and predominates at this point.

Here is an example of how an evaluator should try to help a patient circumscribe his chief complaint.

A 34-year-old secretary came to the clinic with the following complaints:

PATIENT: I have had several problems which I would like to solve. In the last three years I had two unsuccessful relationships with men. I find that I have a tendency to be controlled, yet they complain that it is I who try to control them. This problem has led to the end of my relationships with them.

EVALUATOR: Who ended it, you or they?

PATIENT: They did. The first one actually had said that he was unhappy to terminate our relationships because he liked me very much. He said, "Look here, I cannot see any point in going on because I don't want to be involved with someone who leaves me no breathing space. Everything I do you want to control. I can't take it any longer."

EVALUATOR: And how did you feel?

PATIENT: I felt anxious and sad. These symptoms I also want to get rid of, but before I tell you about these symptoms, I want to add that what actually made me call and make an appointment to see you has to do with recognizing that I am developing this "controlling or being controlled" tendency with my current boyfriend, Mike, whom I like very much, and I would hate to lose him.

EVALUATOR: Any other difficulties?

PATIENT: Yes, I don't get along very well with women. Here is an example of what I mean: I had an opportunity to live with two other women in a nice apartment in Cambridge, but I turned them down because I don't like the idea of having roommates. So I now live in a rooming house all by myself and I pay a much higher rent.

EVALUATOR: Anything else?

PATIENT: Coming back to these symptoms, I think that my feeling anxious upsets my stomach. I haven't had much appetite, I lost some weight, and I don't sleep very well. I am restless at night. I wake up several times during the night and I keep on thinking about all these difficulties.

EVALUATOR: Have you seen a doctor about these physical symptoms, the stomach upset, the loss of weight, and so on?

PATIENT: No, I haven't.

EVALUATOR: Well, first things first. We must have a look at all these physical symptoms. Although you may be right that they are associated with your anxieties, nevertheless they may also be due to other causes. Thus I shall make an appointment for you to be examined in the medical clinic. Is this all right?

PATIENT: Oh, yes. That is OK.

EVALUATOR: But let us return to your complaints. You have symptoms psychological and physical, you have difficulties about control with your boyfriends, and you don't get along very well with women. Now, which is the most important problem?

PATIENT: They are all important. I want help in overcoming them all.

EVALUATOR: I understand that that is what you want, but if we were to help you only with *one* of these difficulties, which one would you choose? Which one would you give top priority for its resolution?

PATIENT: It is difficult to choose.

EVALUATOR: I know, but do try to answer my questions.

PATIENT: Maybe they are all interrelated.

EVALUATOR: Maybe they are, but maybe they are not. So which one would you choose?

PATIENT: . . . OK. Come to think of it, I would say that the problem with my boyfriends is the most important. The anxiety and the sadness I can tolerate, even if they prevailed. The problems that I have with women in a sense I have avoided by living by myself, so if I have to choose I'd pick the issue with men.

Although the evaluator intervenes by offering to make an appointment at the medical clinic to investigate the patient's physical symptoms, he nevertheless gives her an opportunity to make a choice as to the one problem she wants to concentrate on. The patient is able to select what in her opinion is her top priority. In this sense she fulfills nicely the first selection criterion for STAPP.

Patients who are not good STAPP candidates invariably tend to present a variety of complaints in a very diffuse way, and, despite the efforts of the evaluator, they continue to persist in wanting relief for *all* their problems. One is usually struck by their inability to compromise and their considerable rigidity, which is probably due to their excessive narcissistic needs.

There is, however, one set of circumscribed symptoms which should not be confused with what has been said up to now, and their presence should not constitute evidence that the patient's who present them are good candidates for STAPP. I am referring, of course, to fixed delusions. A specific hypochondriacal fear, or a paranoid idea, for example, may at face value be similar to neurotic circumscribed complaints, but there are two basic attitudes of the patient which can easily help us differentiate between the two sets of symptoms. The first of these has to do with the helplessness with which sicker patients deal with their delusions. They seem to be totally at the mercy of their symptoms. The second deals with the absence of affect. The obvious difference lies in the nature of the conflicts underlying these fixed delusions. These conflicts point to a basic weakness in the patient's character structure and reveal evidence that very serious interpersonal difficulties have existed which gave rise to chaotic life situations.

In case some doubt may still persist in the mind of the evaluator as far as the first selection criterion is concerned, he can usually rely on our second criterion, which will invariably come to his rescue and will help him evaluate properly the patient's overall personality organization.

HISTORY OF ONE MEANINGFUL RELATIONSHIP DURING THE PATIENT'S EARLY CHILDHOOD

I must admit that at first this criterion created a great deal of confusion among those who attempted to select appropriate STAPP candidates because of lack of specifications as to what constitutes a "meaningful" relationship.

I have used the terms "altruistic" and "give and take" as synonyms with the word "meaningful," but obviously further clarification is necessary. I shall try, therefore, to present some general guidelines as to what is meant by this term and then to give specific examples which may help dispell any confusion which is likely to be encountered.

The word "meaningful" involves offering something as well as receiving something in return, but the nature of what is given and what is taken should be specified. During the earliest period of the development of the mother–child relationship, the child takes everything from the mother. He takes food, he takes love, he takes all he can get. In this passive way the child depends on the mother and other members of the family for his safety and his security. Pleasure is the result of all this taking, and when this provision of care is threatened with interrruption, pain is promptly experienced and is usually expressed by the tears or screams so familiar to everyone.

The importance of the early mother–child interactions on humans are all well known and will not be discussed here. Suffice it to say that at some time the child's curiosity and need to explore, which sooner or later make their appearance, begin to come in conflict with this need to receive. Bowlby's dramatic description of the young child's exploratory ventures away from the mother emphasizes the need to become independent and separate, yet at the same time to conserve the basic feelings of safety which have existed up to that time. The child is viewed as being attached to the mother by an elastic string which can be stretched appropriately or recoiled in case of danger, or at a time when she makes a move to get up or depart. If the threat of separation immediately brings to the child the need to take, then the newly discovered pleasures of exploration must quickly be abandoned or some other kind of compromise must be established. The possibility of giving something to the mother in return instead of taking all from her is discovered as a new way of keeping her close. Thus a novel way of dealing with this dilemma is found. A precious toy is offered as a token of love and is sacrificed so that the love from the mother and the taking from her can be maintained. These early beginnings of self-sacrifice are compensated with a smile or a kiss and become the early signs of the establishment of a give-and-take relationship. The child has learned to reciprocate the love which he has been receiving.

Altruism is the result of the give-and-take interaction and is, in this most sophisticated way, the logical extension of the early mother–child transaction. One learns that by sacrificing something important, something cherished, he will get in return the love which he needs. This tendency, which at times may go to the extreme of sacrificing one's own life, is viewed by our society as one of the noblest human virtues. Later on in life the pleasure–pain aspects of this early dyadic relationship become replaced to a large extent by an exchange of ideas and feelings. This cognitive and affective component becomes one of the most important aspects of interpersonal exchange, and it is this component which must be assessed when one scrutinizes these early relationships during the evaluation interview.

Thus the ability to have one such meaningful relationship with another person denotes a considerable degree of maturity. Flexibility of feelings of self-sacrifice, without necessarily going to extremes, points to the attainment by the patient of a considerable degree of individuation and a sense of independence.

However, the realities of the outside world compel one, sooner or later, in order to be able to maintain one's own sense of independence and identity, to begin making choices and to learn to arrive at unpleasant decisions. The realization that "what is bad is always true," as Goethe put it, helps one pursue the truth, painful as it may be. Exposure to the fickle inconsistencies and unpredictable behavioral patterns of human relations, with the resulting frustrations, teaches one very quickly how to cope with sudden surprises, unexpected separations, failures to live up to expectations, and finally prepares one to face the ultimate and most painful crisis of all—the loss of a loved one.

Thus the individual who in his early life is prepared to make sacrifices for the sake of someone else, and who is willing to take risks and deny himself some pleasure, learns very quickly through this experience how to deal with people.

He passes the vital test which, like a vaccine, immunizes him for the rest of his life and gives him a prototype for handling future relations with others that follow a similar pattern.

On a more practical level, as the evaluator is scrutinizing the patient's early relationships during the history taking, one of the best questions to ask is whether the patient had *one good friend*. He must not expect, of course, a yes-or-no answer but must require a specific example of the existence of such a friendship. Such a friendship is an excellent indicator that the patient has had a "meaningful relationship" earlier in his life. Here is an example of someone who does not fulfill the second selection criterion:

A 24-year-old single female model who complained of asthmatic attacks described in glowing terms her relationship with her grandmother while she was growing up. Her mother, who had divorced her husband soon after the patient was born, married her lover, and the young child was brought up by her paternal grandmother who referred to her son as "weak" and to his ex-wife as "devoid of education, manners, and culture." The following exchange took place with the evaluator at this point:

PATIENT: My grandmother loved me. She took care of me. She gave me everything I wanted. You will say as others do that she spoiled me, but this is not true, because I was also very good to her.

EVALUATOR: What do you mean?

PATIENT: I did exactly what she wanted.

EVALUATOR: Can you give me an example?

PATIENT: Of course. You see, I was a good child. I never gave my grandmother cause for concern. I never spoke back to her. I never crossed her. I—

EVALUATOR (*interrupting*): Did you enjoy doing all these things?

PATIENT: Oh, yes!

EVALUATOR: Well, if this is the case, did you do anything to please your grandmother which you did not enjoy doing?

PATIENT: Oh, no, no, no. I always enjoyed it.

EVALUATOR: Let me put it differently. Did you do anything that you disliked in order to make your grandmother happy, just to please her?

PATIENT: Of course not! You don't understand. My grandmother never wanted me to do anything that I disliked doing. She called me her "little princess." She used to say, "My little adorable child should never raise her little finger. She should never do anything for anyone else." It was good advice! I never did anything for someone else and I never felt such a need. Actually, on second thought, by modeling I give pleasure to a lot of people.

EVALUATOR: I see. Tell me, does that make you happy?

PATIENT: Yes, it does. I love to wear beautiful new clothes. I look good in them. My grandmother always admires me. I work hard but I like my work.

EVALUATOR: Well, that is not exactly what I had in mind. Let me ask you a question. Would you do anything to please someone else?

PATIENT (*reflecting*): To be perfectly honest with you, doctor . . . the answer is no.

EVALUATOR: Not even your grandmother?

PATIENT: Oh, I see. You don't seem to understand. My grandmother would not want me to sacrifice anything for her. It's against her teachings. She wants me to be happy, and I'm perfectly happy. These attacks of asthma, I'm sure, are due to allergies, although the doctor who referred me to your clinic thinks that they are due to an emotional upset. I am unaware of any such upset.

EVALUATOR: Let me ask you one last question. Do you have or have you ever had a steady boyfriend or a close girlfriend?

PATIENT: That's a funny question. Steady, of course not. Boyfriends? Yes, many. I'm going out with three fellows right now. I like them all. They amuse me, they entertain me, they take me out to nice places. They don't ask for anything in return. Oh, a little sex here and there, but I enjoy that too. I know that you'll say I'm spoiled. Everyone says that. Whatever you want to call it is your business. Any more questions?

EVALUATOR: No, thank you.

Narcissism reigns supreme!

It should be emphasized at this point, however, that a failure to develop one meaningful relationship with another person, and therefore failure to fulfill the second selection criterion for STAPP, is usually due to an early fixation most likely caused by one, a combination of several, or all of the following factors: narcissism, passivity, dependence, sadomasochism, and acting-out tendencies. Thus every evaluator must pay special attention during the history taking to determining the presence of these personality traits, which, if they predominate, will not qualify the patient to receive STAPP.

The ability of the patient to have one meaningful relationship with another person is on occasion difficult to demonstrate. In such a case a second interview, preferably with another evaluator of the opposite sex, may help clarify the situation. Sometimes patients who have had a good relationship with a member of their family who died tend to repress the painful memories associated with this loss and give the false impression during the history taking of not having experienced such a give-and-take interaction.

Another way to test whether or not the patient fulfills the second criterion is to check the manner in which he relates with the evaluator during the interview.

The negative aspects of the search for "one meaningful relationship" have been emphasized up to now. Here is an example of a patient who fulfills this criterion for selection:

A 21-year-old male college student was asked during his evaluation if he had one good friend in his childhood. He responded as follows:

PATIENT: Oh, yes. When I was seven years old John and I were inseparable. He lived very close by and many times he would come and spend the weekend with me. My mother was very fond of him and felt sorry for him.

EVALUATOR: Why?

PATIENT: You see, his father was an alcoholic or drank too much. He had a violent temper. They never invited me to their house because of his father. John was very apologetic about it. His mother, on the other hand, was very nice.

EVALUATOR: So, what was your friendship like?

PATIENT: Well, we used to play soccer. John was poor. He had no toys. When we played soccer it was always with my soccer ball or one of the other kids'. I remember how happy John was when he had received a soccer ball as a Christmas present from his uncle. He showed it to me with great pride and he was planning to use it the next time that we were planning to play the following week. But when the time came John came to my house early. He was crying. When I asked him what was the matter. He said that he had accidentally broken his father's favorite beer mug—one that his father had brought back from Germany after World War II. It seems that his father was furious. He had been drinking, so as a punishment he took a kitchen knife and tore John's soccer ball to ribbons. John was very upset about it and he felt humiliated when he was thinking of how to explain all this to the other kids that afternoon. He wanted me to tell them that he was sick just as an excuse. I said to him, "No, John, you are taking the easy way out if you don't show up. But I am going to help you." So I want up to my room, where I had two soccer balls—one was also brand-new and the other an old one. I said to myself, Well, I'll give John the old one, but I thought that the other kids would have expected John to have a new one, so I took my own new one and gave it to John. He didn't want to accept it but I convinced him. He was very happy. I was a bit said to give it up but his happiness made me happy.

A seven-year-old who makes a sacrifice for his friend certainly passes with flying colors the test of our second criterion.

FLEXIBLE INTERACTION WITH THE EVALUATOR AND ABILITY TO EXPRESS FEELINGS OPENLY DURING THE INTERVIEW

If the patient has had a meaningful relationship during his early life, he should have learned to face new situations and to interact flexibly with people. Thus he should be capable of relating well with the evaluator and should be expected to be able to express feelings openly, appropriately, and freely during the evaluation.

The nature of the feelings which one has access to during the interview should preferably be varied, but the presence of anger should not be interpreted as signifying that the patient is not a good candidate. Negative feelings, such as anger, sadness, or fear, if appropriate to a realistic situation and if experienced with moderation, point to good reality testing and indicate the presence of a strong personality organization.

Flexibility also implies an ability to adjust quickly to a new situation, necessitating the appropriate expression of different kinds of feelings. If, for example, a patient has felt sad about an event in his life which required such a response, he should be able to express a similar feeling when he is talking about it during his evaluation interview.

In my experience, one of the pitfalls commonly encountered during the psychological evaluation has to do with the tendency of the evaluators not to scrutinize very carefully their own interaction with the patient so as not to encourage the early development of transference feelings. Athough this is true as far as seriously disturbed patients are concerned, it does not apply to good STAPP candidates. If anything, the contrary is the rule with such individuals. Transference feelings should be talked about as soon as possible, because the early utilization of such feelings is an important technical requirement for this kind of treatment (as will be discussed more extensively in later chapters). Here is an example:

A 27-year-old male accountant had made an appointment in the clinic one month in advance because of certain difficulties which he encountered at work. He arrived 15 minutes early for his evaluation interview. The evaluator, who had had to attend an unscheduled administrative meeting, called the clinic to say that he would be delayed. He actually arrived 10 minutes late, apologized to the patient, and was in the process of beginning the interview when the patient interrupted him to say that he had felt annoyed while waiting for him. The following exchange took place:

EVALUATOR: You see, it was an unavoidable emergency.

PATIENT: I do understand, don't get me wrong, but I also consider punctuality a very important character trait. I am always on time and I expect the same from others.

EVALUATOR: Yes, of course. Can you tell me a little more how you feel about this situation?

PATIENT: I am an accountant and I am a perfectionist. I do a good job. I spend much of my time dealing with details. I work around the clock, and I am punctual, as I have told you already. You see, I made this appointment long in advance. I came early to be sure that I found a parking place. I wasted a lot of time. I understand that you are busy, but so am I.

EVALUATOR: So, I see that you're angry at me.

PATIENT: Not angry, just annoyed.

EVALUATOR: All right, then, annoyed.

PATIENT: That's true. I thought that it was appropriate for me to tell you how I feel, otherwise I wouldn't be honest. I don't want to give the impression that I am intolerant. It is also possible that am a little too rigid, and that these difficulties at work which brought me to this clinic may stem from this attitude of mine. I just wanted to have these feelings out of the way right from the start. I am prepared to examine and to question my behavior, and I am ready to work hard. I do accept your apology and I am now ready to answer your questions.

This forthright presentation on the part of the patient, which relates to a realistic situation, is evidence of considerable strength and points to his ability to express his feelings appropriately—to the right person, at the right place, and at the right time.

Something should also be said at this point about the nature of the interaction with the evaluator in terms of the patient's overall behavior, his facial expression, his bodily movements, his posture, his eye contact, and his general appearance.

The nonverbal aspects of the interaction between evaluator and patient may be considered to be obvious, yet, because of this, little attention is usually paid to this important aspect of the interview. The inappropriate smile, for example, may indicate much more to the evaluator than a long description of various events and circumstances on the part of the patient. In reference to such elaborate descriptions of details instead of feelings, one should keep in mind the observations of the French psychoanalysts Marty, de M'Uzan, and David, who have called this kind of thinking the *pensée opératoire*. This utilitarian way of thinking coupled with a poor fantasy life, a tendency to take impulsive action, and an inability to use appropriate words to describe feelings, I have called "alexithymia." In our experience as well as in that of other investigators, "alexithymia" occurs quite often in patients suffering from psychosomatic diseases, but it may also be found in individuals who are not medically ill (Nemiah & Sifneos, 1970; Nemiah, 1977; Taylor, 1984).

Observations of this kind should be made during the evaluation interview. Alexithymic patients not only show the above-mentioned characteristics but also tend to assume rigid postures, show inappropriate facial expressions, and avoid looking at the interviewer. At times they are inappropriately dressed and usually tend to arouse countertransference feelings of boredom (Sifneos *et al.,* 1977).

Alexithymia seems to be a deficiency in the area of affects in the same way as Korsakoff's patients have problems with their memory. Although the alexithymic patient is able to be aware of emotions and to think, he seems unable to connect any thoughts with his emotions. Thus he has an inability to experience feelings—a *feeling* being defined as "a biological emotion *plus* the thoughts which accompany it."

Although the etiology of this phenomenon is unknown at the

present time, it has been hypothesized that neuroanatomical or neurophysiological defects in the area of the limbic system and its connection with the neocortex, between right and left hemispheres or both, may be responsible for alexithymic characteristics. It has also been thought that these deficiencies may be due to arrests in emotional development during childhood, or to massive regressions caused by environmental onslaughts. Other possibilities involve sociocultural factors or excessive use of psychological defense mechanisms such as denial or regression.

Observations, then, as to the presence or absence of these alexithymic characteristics should be kept in mind during the evaluation session while the interviewer is investigating whether or not the patient fulfills the third criterion. It should be quite obvious from this discussion not only that an alexithymic individual is a poor candidate for STAPP but also that if these difficulties are due to biological defects, psychodynamic psychotherapy of brief or long-term duration should be contraindicated for the patient.

PSYCHOLOGICAL SOPHISTICATION—ABOVE-AVERAGE INTELLIGENCE AND PSYCHOLOGICAL MINDEDNESS

Although, at first, we were primarily interested in assessing the patient's intellectual endowments as demonstrated by specific achievements, as time went by we started to pay more and more attention to another aspect of the patient's character traits which involves a certain degree of psychological mindedness. The two together are referred to as "psychological sophistication." This term implies a familiarity with psychological constructs; it refers to an ability to deal with conflicting states, to tolerate paradoxical situations, and to exhibit behavioral patterns appropriate to such occurrences. For example, a patient who is convinced that a stomach pain which occurs whenever he has a fight with his supervisor at work must be due exclusively to physical factors, and who refuses to investigate the possibility that psychological issues may be associated with it, does not show evidence of psychological sophistication.

Furthermore, we like to document above-average intelligence on the basis of the patient's performance at work or academic achievement. The evaluator should be able to make a rough guess of the patient's IQ and to predict whether or not during the course

of the therapy he would be able to utilize his intelligence construc-
tively to help himself overcome his problem.

One of the reasons we have paid so much attention to the patient's having above-average intellectual capabilities has to do with
the discovery that the cognitive component of STAPP, as evidenced
in the patient's ability to problem-solve, played an important role
in the successful results which have been obtained in long-term
follow-up interviews (more about this will be discussed in Chapter
13).

I do not want to give the impression, however, that the patient's psychological sophistication should be equated with his social class or his educational background. Here is an example:

A 37-year-old fruit vendor complained of a phobia which kept
him in the confines of Boston's West End, an area of the city which
was considered to be a slum and whose population was in the process of relocation. He was apprehensive because he was told by his
mother that the relocation office social worker had found a new
apartment for them in the suburbs and that, in the near future, they
would have to move. This precipitated a crisis for the patient, who
then came to the clinic for help.

The patient was a tall, friendly man, and a warm smile usually
appeared on his face. He was totally illiterate and indicated that he
worked for his father as a vendor of fruits and vegetables in the
West End. When his father wanted to open a new shop in another
part of the city and asked him to take over the supervision of the
new shop, the patient refused, claiming that he was afraid to cross
the street which in his mind constituted the boundary line between
the West End and the rest of Boston. His father was angry with him
and decided to run the new shop himself, leaving the old shop
the responsibility of his son.

The patient was visibly anxious when he recounted his fear of
moving, but then he added:

PATIENT: There's something else, doc. I don't know if it's important,
but I thought that I should talk about it. . . .
EVALUATOR: Go on.
PATIENT: Well, it has to do with my mother. (*Hesitating*) . . . See,
when I get close to Cambridge Street, you know the street which
I'm afraid to cross, I start hearing my mother's voice calling me.
EVALUATOR (*startled*): You hear voices?

PATIENT: Oh, no, doc! I'm not crazy, you know. No, it's just like this. It's my mother's voice inside my head. It's my thinking, see! It's that I think that she's calling me.

EVALUATOR: And what does she say in your thoughts?

PATIENT: Well, she says, "Mario, come home," and then I ask, "Is father home?" "No," she says, "the house is all yours and I've cooked a good meal for you." So you see, doc, I can't cross the street because there's something pulling me back and making me go home.

EVALUATOR: So, you are not afraid of crossing the street; it is that something pulls you back.

PATIENT: Gee, doc! I never thought of it this way, but you're right.

EVALUATOR: Well, it is you who put it this way. But then you say that you ask her about your father. Why do you do that?

PATIENT: Well, I don't feel like rushing back to my house when he's around. He always has something to complain about. When my mother and I are alone (*smiling*) we have such a good time, Doc!

EVALUATOR: So, your father has also something to do with your trouble?

PATIENT: Well, they both do. You see, I've been thinking about all this. My dad's pushing me to go away. He wants me to take over the other shop and to leave the West End. My mother wants me to stay home. So, you see, doc, I'm having a problem, but this fear makes it impossible for me to leave.

EVALUATOR: Well, as we have seen, it's not the fear that stops you but rather the wish to be alone with your mother. When your father is around, he stops the good time you have with your mother.

PATIENT (*smiling*): You're smart, doc. That's really it, I guess. So what do you think? Is there hope for me?

EVALUATOR: What do *you* think?

PATIENT: Yeah. I guess so. If it's all in my head I must be able to help myself.

The dynamics of this case are obvious. What is striking is the simple and straightforward way in which the patient is aware of his problem and his realization that he has the potential to resolve it. In his simple way he must be considered as being highly sophisticated psychologically.

In reference to his case it should be mentioned that as a result of offering psychotherapy to a group of patients of low socioeconomic and educational level who were facing forced relocation as a result of urban renewal, we discovered that a considerable number of these individuals were good STAPP candidates and did very well when they were offered this therapy. It was evident therefore that patients who were intelligent and psychologically minded, as well as fulfilling the other criteria for selection for STAPP, did not have to be well educated or to come from a social class which was once thought to respond well to psychotherapeutic interventions. One should emphasize, however, that a certain explanatory statement should be made by the evaluator as to what is expected of the patient and of how the treatment proceeds. This must be done in a simple, straightforward way, and psychiatric jargon should by all means be avoided.

The question of superior intelligence presents some problems because it carries with it a certain element of a value judgment. For example, our fourth selection criterion created some difficulty when it was discussed with a group of psychiatrists in Oslo, Norway, where I was engaged in setting up a research study of short-term psychotherapy a few years ago. What bothered my Norwegian colleagues was the potential stigma associated with someone's not being able to fulfill this fourth criterion. One way in which they were able to resolve this problem was to inquire into the patient's educational achievements. For example, if he passed his high school equivalency, the patient was considered to be of above-average intelligence. Although this may be practical in Norway, I do not recommend it as a good rule of thumb in the United States, where high school educational standards vary enormously. Thus the effort should be made by the evaluator to try to determine whether the patient fulfills this criterion by collecting the necessary evidence during the history taking so as to be able to assess the patient's overall intelligence adequately, without having to rely on psychological tests. If this is not possible, however, then psychological tests should be given.

MOTIVATION FOR CHANGE

The fifth STAPP selection criterion is associated with the sense of dissatisfaction experienced by the patient about his behavior patterns and with the willingness on his part to make a concentrated effort to alter them. Thus, motivation *for change* should not be confused with motivation for symptom relief, which implies more a need to remove or change painful feelings. In contrast to a passive state of being, motivation for change implies an activity on the part of the patient, which denotes that he is willing to take a responsibility for the therapeutic task and to rely on his own resources rather than to depend on the therapist.

I have defined "motivation for change" as "a problem-solving process." As such, it is a powerful force within an individual that leads to action. Furthermore, it is associated with an individual's creative process and his ability to be curious, to be inspired, to discover, and to invent. Invariably, creativity and motivation go hand in hand, not only in those aspects already mentioned but also in various forms of their expression.

Each individual who is motivated to change his lifestyle has an opportunity to use his talents effectively and to emerge from adversity a freer and happier human being.

We have studied the patient's motivation for change extensively and have discovered that it is not only an important selection criterion for STAPP but also a prognostic guideline of STAPP's successful outcome.

For example, in one of our first studies, 25 patients had received STAPP and 10 had received brief anxiety-suppressive psychotherapy, all having achieved successful results as stated by both the patients and their therapists. In 31 of these patients, or 88%, they were rated as having had "fair" to "excellent" motivation for change using a 7-point scale consisting of criteria for assessing motivation. On the other hand, of the 5 patients who received STAPP and the 15 who received brief anxiety-suppressive therapy and who did poorly in their therapy, 12, or 60%, were considered to be unmotivated to change (Sifneos, 1968 b).

Because of its prognostic value, and from our overall clinical experience, we decided that motivation for change was probably the most important of all the criteria we have used for selection of patients to receive STAPP. We have, therefore, developed seven additional criteria to evaluate motivation for change. These are the following:

1. *Willingness to participate actively in the psychiatric evaluation.* What

is expected in reference to this criterion has to do with the patients' ability to get engaged in an active interaction with the evaluator in order to learn how to problem-solve. Although the patients may not exactly know what is expected of them the first time they visit a mental health professional, they should not expect to remain passive and wait for all the questioning to emanate from the evaluator. On the contrary, spontaneous contributions in the form of memories, fantasies, or episodes in their lives which add to the establishment of a clear picture of the development of their psychological difficulties are invaluably helpful, and this information sets the tone of what is likely to take place during STAPP.

2. *Honesty in reporting about oneself.* The ability to give an honest and truthful account of their emotional conflicts, difficult as it may be, demonstrates that the patients are capable of presenting themselves in a true light and that they are not trying to hide or pretend to give a good impression of themselves so as to please their evaluators.

3. *Ability to recognize that the symptoms are psychological in origin.* A degree of psychological sophistication is an indication that the patients are aware, even if this is unclear, that emotional conflicts are an underlying cause of their symptoms, and that they do not rush to attribute them to physical reasons. Although a certain degree of instruction about the nature of psychotherapy is necessary with unsophisticated patients, if a patient possesses some insights, then the length of the treatment is likely to be shortened.

4. *Introspection and curiosity.* Self-inquisitiveness, whether due to curiosity or not, is a helpful asset which will facilitate the task of the therapist. It is hoped that as the treatment progresses, the patients' curiosity will be further aroused by the therapist's demonstration of peculiar patterns of behavior, past–present links, paradoxical clarifications, and so on.

5. *Openness to new ideas.* A certain ability to explore new ideas and to experiment with different behavioral attitudes again demonstrates not only a constructive and active curiosity but also intelligence, openness, and flexibility, personality traits that will help in the task of problem solving, one of the most important technical aspects of STAPP.

6. *Realistic expectations of the results of the treatment.* This criterion emphasizes the ability of the patients to assess and to test reality

correctly. Grandiose or unrealistic expectations of the therapeutic outcome denote a certain degree of narcissism or a lack of flexibility, which would be factors that might complicate or even interfere with its successful completion.

7. *Willingness to make a reasonable sacrifice.* If the patients are to be truly motivated to change, they should be willing to make a reasonable and tangible sacrifice so as to achieve a successful outcome. For example, they should be able to compromise in matters such as an appointment time or a fee for their therapy. Recently, when we started to use videotaping of STAPP, we expected that patients would resist our requests, yet to our surprise we found that not only were they willing to cooperate but they actually liked the idea of having their therapy become a model to help train therapists in this short-term modality and to help investigate its value.

A forced-choice questionnaire containing all these seven criteria is used to give a rating to motivation for change. Thus a score of 7 is considered "excellent" motivation, 6 is "good," 5 is "fair," and 4 is "questionable." Anyone with a score below 4 is considered to be "unmotivated."

In two more recent studies, 42 patients who came to the psychiatric clinic of the Beth Israel Hospital in Boston and were treated by 15 therapists had their motivation for change evaluated during their first, fourth, and eighth interviews of psychotherapy. It appeared that in 33, or 78%, the motivation increased or stayed at the same level, while it decreased in only 9 patients (Sifneos, 1971).

Finally, out of a homogeneous group of 53 fairly disturbed patients treated by 36 therapists, two-thirds of those whose scores on motivation were high during their evaluation maintained this high level after the end of their therapy (Sifneos, 1978). These patients were considered to have achieved successful therapeutic results as rated by a questionnaire which included 12 outcome criteria (to be described in a later chapter). Thus it again appears that motivation for change not only is basic for STAPP patients but also seems to play an important role in the successful psychotherapy of more severely disturbed individuals.

The absence of motivation for change or its decrease during the course of psychotherapy should be viewed as a serious sign because it indicates an absence of anxiety, which acts as an important motivating factor.

The ability to tolerate a certain amount of this unpleasant feeling indicates considerable strength of character. An example here may be appropriate:

A 27-year-old musician wanted to resolve his difficulties with his friends which clearly stemmed from an ambivalent relationship with his father. He was rated as having "good" motivation for change, but by the fourth interview his rating had dropped to 4, which is considered "questionable." What had happened was that his father offered to finance a trip to Austria for him to study music, with the proviso that he break off his engagement to a girl of whom the father disapproved. The relationship with his fiancée was considered to be a good one, and it was an indication that he was willing to stand on his own ground and not give in to his father's authoritarian wishes. All this had been discussed during the first few sessions, and the patient was in agreement with this assessment. The therapist was surprised, therefore, to hear that the patient was seriously considering accepting his father's offer that he should give up his fiancée and stop his therapy. Although this was discussed at some length during the fifth interview, and despite the fact that both therapist and patient were in agreement with the formulation that his difficulties with his father which played a role in bringing him to the clinic had not been resolved, and that the patient's acceptance of his father's offer would perpetuate the difficulties, the patient nevertheless decided to accept it.

It was of interest that he returned to the clinic one year later stating that the problem with his father was still present, that his year in Vienna was not as successful as he had thought it would be, and that he had missed both his fiancée and his therapy. He admitted that he had made a serious mistake. Would the clinic give him "a second chance," he asked. The answer was yes. During his second therapeutic endeavor, his motivation for change was maintained high throughout the course of therapy, and he was able to make a successful resolution of his psychological problems over a brief period of time.

Our criteria for selection of STAPP patients have served us well over the years. They have provided us with a way to avoid the interminable and so familiar discussions about the patient's psycho pathology, while at the same time they offer the advantage of a practical set of parameters which can easily be assessed during the evaluation of the patient.

Because of these advantages, I think that all kinds of psycho-therapies of short and long duration should specify clear and distinct criteria for selection. If this were to take place, a big step toward evaluating a variety of psychotherapeutic interventions would have been taken, making the eventual validation of their efficacy a much easier task.

CHAPTER 4

The Psychological Evaluation Process: Part III

It should be made clear from the outset that it is not my intention to present a fragmented picture of the evaluation process by dividing it artificially into three distinct parts. I do not want to give the impression that certain tasks performed by the evaluator are independent of the overall continuous process of the psychological evaluation. The information obtained about the patient's chief complaint and the history of the patient's psychological development must blend smoothly with the assessment of the criteria for selection for STAPP and with the establishment of a specific therapeutic focus.

THE PSYCHODYNAMIC FORMULATION AND THE ASSESSMENT OF SPECIFIC PREDISPOSING VULNERABILITY

The Therapeutic Focus

On the basis of the information amassed from the patient, somewhere during the evaluation interview the evaluator must arrive at a psychodynamic formulation of the patient's psychological problem. This formulation must take into consideration all the specific predisposing factors which make the patient vulnerable to various hazardous situations. This formulation must also select a therapeutic focus which crystallizes the specific psychological conflicts underlying the patient's psychological problem that must be resolved during the psychotherapy.

The therapeutic focus must be communicated to the patient, and an effort should be made to obtain his cooperation and his agreement. This mutual interaction, which usually takes place at the end of the first or, at the latest, during the second interview, is referred to as the "contract" between the two protagonists. The agreement on the therapeutic focus as established in the "contract" becomes the central point on which the future therapeutic work will concentrate.

In a psychiatric clinic or mental health agency the evaluator and the therapist are usually different individuals. If this is the case, the therapist must repeat the evaluation process and must arrive at the same or possibly a slightly modified focus. In private practice, on the other hand, this is not necessary since the therapist is also the evaluator; thus this procedure becomes greatly simplified. An example of this point may clarify this somewhat theoretical presentation of the evaluation process:

A 24-year-old single female college graduate student complained of anxiety following the end of her relationship with her boyfriend with whom she had been living for the past year. She was aware that she was responsible for the difficulties between the two of them, which led to their separation, and attributed this to her progressive dissatisfaction with her boyfriend. This disenchantment with a man whom she had liked a great deal had occurred with other men with whom she had relations in the past and constituted a repetitive pattern which invariably made the end of the relationships inevitable. When she was asked to describe exactly when she became aware of the change in her attitude toward her boyfriend, she readily told of her need to make impossible demands on him and her dissatisfaction with his inability to meet these unrealistic expectations. Again she pointed out that this pattern had existed in her previous relations with men whom she was fond of and described her irritation with them as similar to her feelings about her current ex-boyfriend.

During the history taking, it became clear to the evaluator that this young woman's attitude was associated with her relationship with her father, to whom she was very much attached, and who had reciprocated her feelings until the time when her brother was born when she was nine years old. She remembered clearly feeling very resentful and jealous when her father praised her brother, and she recalled how she felt very angry at her brother, wishing he would "disappear." This resentment was seen as having been displaced on the various boyfriends during her adolescence and contributed to making the patient vulnerable to these inevitable separations from men. In the evaluator's opinion this vulnerability was considered to be the specific factor which predisposed the patient to repeat the pattern of her relation with her father and brother in her relationships with other men. It was decided then that this should become the therapeutic focus for her STAPP, and this was communicated to her. She readily agreed to explore her feelings in this area of psychological difficulties, and the practical arrangements for her treatment began at this point.

This psychodynamic theoretical formulation by the evaluator of the patient's difficulties is intimately connected with an understanding of the specific predisposing factors which explain the patient's psychological problem and which lead to the establishment of the therapeutic focus.

Focalization

The establishment of a dynamic focus, which, according to Strupp, involves "the problem of gathering and organizing therapeutically relevant information" (Strupp, 1984) and around which revolves short-term dynamic psychotherapy, is accepted by most investigators in this field as a basic prerequisite for this form of psychiatric treatment. Furthermore, there is general consensus that unresolved Oedipal conflicts, grief reactions, and certain problems relating to loss and separation issues are the foci which, when they are resolved, give rise to the best therapeutic results.

Various centers of investigation have done systematic research on patients whose therapeutic focus was identical so as to obtain a homogeneous population. For example, Horowitz and his colleagues have studied patients who faced the loss of a loved one (Horowitz, 1984), and by emphasizing the importance of paying special attention to personality styles, they tailor-make, so to speak, the therapy to deal with them.

Other workers in the field have dealt with focalizations by letting the patient select his own focus rather than by having the therapist select what in his opinion was the best area to work on. Gillieron, in Lausanne, emphasizing the importance of the therapeutic setting (*le cadre*), which he defines as the confines of the therapy in temporal and spatial dimensions, and by use of free association manages to force the patient to establish his own focus (Gillieron, 1983). Mann, in Boston, using the time-limited therapeutic approach of 12 interviews, also helps the patient develop the "central issue" around which his therapy will revolve (Mann, 1973). Brusset, in Paris, limits the evaluation to two interviews and manages to negotiate a focus with his patients (Brusset, 1983).

On the other hand, Davanloo, Malan, and Montgrain, in Montreal, London, and Quebec, respectively, themselves establish the focus of their brief psychotherapeutic interventions (Malan, 1976; Montgrain, 1983; Davanloo, personal communication).

In STAPP we also are the ones to choose the appropriate focus upon which to concentrate.

At this point I would like to clarify a misunderstanding which has been created in reference to STAPP, namely, that the unresolved Oedipal focus is the only one to be selected. We do agree with the other investigators that several other foci also can be used in STAPP, but we have indeed selected patients with unresolved Oedipal foci only for research purposes, in an effort to investigate as homogeneous a short-term patient population as possible (Sifneos, 1984).

THE OEDIPAL THERAPEUTIC FOCUS

The underlying psychological conflicts which are usually involved in the therapeutic foci of STAPP patients have to do with Oedipal-genital or triangular-interpersonal interactions. The decision to select patients where an Oedipal focus was clearly identified resulted from several unsuccessfully treated patients chosen for STAPP whose therapeutic focus involved loss or separation from a loved one, and who had developed grief reactions or reactive depressions.

What should be carefully scrutinized, therefore, is the nature of the patterns of separation. If these constitute a way of dealing with Oedipal problems and represent a regressive retreat on the part of the patient in his efforts to deal with such conflicts, then one may still accept such a patient and offer him STAPP. If, on the other hand, the depressive symptomatology denotes a more primitive sensitivity to loss, where certain oral problems predominate and have persisted, then such patients should not be considered as good STAPP candidates because one can predict that serious difficulties are likely to be encountered when early termination of the treatment is discussed with them. Here is an example:

A 25-year-old male engineer was very close to his mother, but he was also happily married and seemed to have good relations with people at work. It was after his mother's sudden death in an automobile accident that he became depressed and sought psychiatric help. During the evaluation, his relations with his mother, his wife, and women in general were scrutinized, but no significant problems were encountered. He was also thought to fulfill the STAPP criteria for selection.

At first the therapy proceeded uneventfully. He made rapid progress in terms of understanding the importance of his attachments for his mother. He was only partially able to express feelings of ambivalence about her death, however, and preferred to talk at length about his positive feelings for her. After some weeks, he started to feel better, and his depression seemed to have improved. At this point the therapist thought that termination should be considered and he communicated this thought to the patient. As soon as the therapist mentioned the possibility of ending psychotherapy, the patient became angry, claiming that he did not want to stop. From then on, despite the therapist's efforts to help the patient work through his hostility, he remained angry. After a few weeks of marked ambivalence highlighted by numerous sarcastic remarks, the patient suddenly announced that he was discontinuing his therapy, stating that he had found a private psychotherapist who was willing to see him "as long as *he* needed to be seen."

It was obvious that this turn of events was disturbing because it pointed to a defective evaluation. How could the patient's dependent needs and excessive sensitivity to separation have been missed during his assessment? Unfortunately, nothing specific could be discovered, and serious doubts about our evaluation sys-

tem started creeping in. By chance, the private therapist to whom
the patient turned was a graduate of our residency training program
who had treated several patients with STAPP and was well acquainted with our evaluation system as well as with our criteria for
selection. When he called the clinic to ask for information about our
findings, he was surprised to hear that we had considered the patient a good STAPP candidate. When asked to amplify his remarks,
he said that in his opinion the patient clearly did not have an Oedipal focus. Furthermore, he thought that this patient's problem was
pregenital and characterological in nature, having to do more with
the early loss and separation of the patient from his grandmother,
who brought him up and who had died when he was four years
old. His subsequent attachment to his mother, which appeared at
face value to be Oedipal and which had misled us during the clinic
evaluation, was really a dependent substitution of his mother for
the dead grandmother. It appeared that the patient's mother had an
important job when the patient was born and did not want to give
it up. Having divorced his father, she asked her widowed mother,
the patient's grandmother, to live with them and take care of her
son. The grandmother readily agreed and took care of the patient,
pampering him and acquiescing to all his demands. When she
died, his mother grudgingly took over the care of the patient. He,
in turn, repressed the painful and ambivalent feelings over the
death of his grandmother. This important information was unavailable to us, possibly having been missed because of the repression,
during our evaluation of the patient. The sudden death of his
mother which brought the patient to the clinic, and at the time was
thought to be a good therapeutic focus to concentrate on, was obviously a repetition of a much greater pregenital trauma which he
had experienced at the time of his grandmother's death. Because we
subsequently had similar difficulties with patients who were selected for STAPP whose therapeutic focus was a "loss of a loved
one," we decided to exclude such individuals from our *research*
study because it was thought that they required a longer time to
deal with their reactions to separation, and for that reason they
were thought not to be ideal STAPP candidates.

This type of difficulty again points to the importance of taking
as systematic a history as possible, where an effort should be made
to discover any pregenital traumata which occurred and which

made an impact on the development of the patient's character and on the symptoms which he subsequently developed.

Our decision to select for STAPP only patients with a clear-cut Oedipal therapeutic focus without a history of earlier pregenital difficulties has been criticized by other investigators who have accepted sicker patients. It was thought that this limitation on our part excluded several patients who might also benefit from brief dynamic psychotherapy.

Our motivation, however, has been to try to delineate as clearly as possible a kind of psychotherapy, such as STAPP, which is very precise and is undoubtedly the treatment of choice for a selected group. The fewer complicating factors that could be specified and investigated, the better. This decision, of course, does not exclude the development of other kinds of short-term dynamic psychotherapy which could be specific for the sicker patients.

Nevertheless, there are a great number of fairly healthy individuals who have clear-cut Oedipal problems and for whom STAPP is the treatment of choice. Furthermore, within the context of the Oedipal focus there are enormous variations in the ways such patients go about dealing with and attempt to solve their Oedipal triangles. Such diversity not only complicates the therapy but also provides the therapist with many new perspectives and makes the therapeutic experience very exciting.

As has already been discussed, the kinds of complaints which are usually related to Oedipal conflicts have to do with the appearance of circumscribed symptoms and/or specific problems in interpersonal relations. Patients with interpersonal difficulties generally do better than those who have developed symptoms. It is possible that once a symptom has appeared and has crystallized out of the patient's efforts to deal with a series of psychological conflicts, it is more difficult to reverse because it provides the patient with a better neurotic solution to his problem than the uncertainty which he experiences whenever he has to deal with people, despite the fact that this symptomatic solution restricts his activities.

The nature of these circumscribed symptoms, however, must also be scrutinized. Symptoms which have already been enumerated and fall within our selection category are phobias, anxieties, mild obsessive-compulsive complaints, and mild depressions (Sifneos, 1985). It should be remembered, however, that a specific paranoid delusion or hypochondriacal preoccupation, although well circumscribed, is not a symptom which is associated with an Oedipal focus and denotes the presence of a much more serious psychopathology.

Although the nature of the transference feelings of STAPP patients for their male or female therapists will be discussed in much greater detail later on, the appearance of such feelings during the evaluation interview has a great deal to do with the assessment of the patient's specific Oedipal focus. From our experience, male or female patients who interact just as well with evaluators of either sex have a better prognosis than those who interact well only with an evaluator of the opposite sex. It is important, therefore, that patients who have difficulty in their interviews with evaluators of the same sex be given an opportunity to be interviewed once more by a second interviewer, preferably of the opposite sex. Here is an example:

A twenty-year-old female factory worker had been rude to the clinic receptionist (a female) as well as to her evaluator, one of our senior social workers (also a female). As a result of the patient's antagonistic attitude, the evaluator had some difficulty in obtaining a good history. When her case was discussed during the intake conference, it was thought that, although an Oedipal focus could be established, the patient was not a good STAPP candidate primarily because she did not fulfill the third selection criterion, namely, "the ability to interact flexibly with the evaluator." Before a final decision was reached, however, it was thought that a second interview with a male evaluator might throw some light on the patient's rudeness, sarcasm, and overall hostility to women. During this interview with the patient a vital bit of information emerged. It appeared that the patient had had an excellent relationship with her mother when she was young. She was an only child; her mother had tried unsuccessfully to conceive for many years and when she finally gave birth to the patient, she was very happy. In terms of the second criterion for selection, namely, "evidence of the existence of one meaningful relationship during the patient's early life," it appeared that her relation with her mother was indeed meaningful and altruistic. For example, the patient related that, when she was four years old, she had given up her cat willingly, although she was very much attached to it, to make her mother, who was allergic to cat hairs, happy. This good relationship ended abruptly, however, after her mother gave birth to another girl five years later. This sister seemed to have instantly become her mother's favorite. "You see," the patient went on bitterly, "my mother liked young babies and I was already a grown child. She replaced me like an old hat. From then on I disliked my mother as well as women in general. My father, on the other hand, who had not played a big role in my life up to that time, became important to me. Actually, in retrospect, I am happy because I discovered Daddy." Her relationship with her father was good, as was, later on, her interaction with her boyfriends. Her competition with women persisted and was what motivated her to seek psychotherapy. The nature of this competition, however, was sexualized. She experienced a feeling of revenge, a feeling of superiority whenever she defeated another woman, using her sexual attraction for men as well as sarcasm and wit as her weapons. She was aware of these problems and was willing at that point to make her "peace with women."

It was clear from this second interview that this patient fulfilled the second selection criterion for STAPP, and, in addition, it was evident that she could relate very well to the male evaluator. It was decided, therefore, that the therapeutic focus should remain an Oedipal one, and every effort should be made to help this patient get some perspective on her competitive feelings toward women. She was treated by a male therapist, and an excellent result was achieved.

At this point it seems to me that one should try to differentiate between individuals who are STAPP candidates and who have had some difficulty in resolving their Oedipal conflict, and ordinary people who have gone through their Oedipal period without developing symptoms and/or interpersonal problems.

We have utilized Malan's (1976a) concept of specific stress, which we call specific internal predisposition (SIP), which in our opinion makes one vulnerable to psychological hazards if during early life one has been unable to resolve successfully a variety of psychological conflicts, in general, and of the specific Oedipal or triangular kind, in particular. Thus, the assessment of each patient's SIP contributes to the general understanding of the patient's psychological difficulties and helps establish clearly the therapeutic focus.

From our observations, female patients who have had a good

relation with their mothers up to the age of four or five years, and, as a result of their subsequent attachment to their fathers, develop competitive feelings for their mothers for which they feel guilty, are the best female STAPP candidates because they have no serious SIP factors to complicate their psychological development.

On the other hand, female patients who, when they made an effort to attach themselves to their fathers, felt that they had been partially rejected because of their fathers' realistic preference for another sibling, seem to have a somewhat more difficult time during their STAPP. If such individuals are able to express their angry feelings openly, they do manage with the help of their therapists to overcome their problem.

In general, male patients have a somewhat easier time since they do not have to switch their affection for their mothers during their Oedipal period. Male patients who had a good relation with their mothers and who are later rejected by them also tend to have somewhat greater difficulty during their STAPP. If, on the other hand, their relations with their mothers had not been so good before the onset of the Oedipal period, their SIP factors create complications which interfere with their treatment and do not make them good candidates for this type of short-term psychotherapy. Here is an example:

A 24-year-old graduate student had described his relationship with his mother in glowing terms. "My mother," he said, "was very special. She was a tease. She was brilliant. She was lovely. She was an artist, and I was interested in painting when I was young. I remember that one of the nicest experiences from my childhood was to look at art books with my mother. I remember that one of her favorite pictures was a painting of a railway stations *La Gare St. La-zare* by Monet, with its hazy blue-gray hues of color." As he was reminiscing about all this, he had a satisfied smile on his face and looked removed from the immediacy of the interview situation. His facial expression soon changed, however, and it became distorted when he started to talk about the birth of his younger brother when he was six years old. This brother was a sickly baby, requiring a great deal of attention from his mother. He remembered that during that time he used to torment his pet dog and was criticized repeatedly by his mother for this sadistic behavior. When asked if he felt jealous of his brother, he seemed to be taken by surprise because he said that he did not remember experiencing such feelings at that time.

It was at the age of 12 when his brother developed polio that he remembered that "all hell broke loose." Both his parents were heartbroken by the turn of events, and he remembered that his parents expected him to act "grown-up" and "not to ask for any special privileges as the elder." On one occasion he remembered his father's words bitterly: "Tim is sick and needs all the attention we can give him. He deserves it and will get it. I know and expect that you will understand that there might not be too much time available for you. It does not mean that we don't love you; it is that you are the elder, you are healthy, and you can face this difficult situation." He spoke rapidly, imitating his father's voice. He said that he was aware of the gravity of the situation, but it was the first time it occurred to him that his brother might die. As to how the family life was going to change, he was unclear.

The crisis occurred one day when he won the first prize in an essay contest at school. It was all about the French Impressionists, and he felt very proud about his achievement. He came home and told his mother of his success, expecting a great deal of praise from her. His mother congratulated him but declined to read the essay at that moment because she was busy preparing his brother's dinner. "Somewhere, deep inside, I was prepared for it," he went on, "but it felt like a stab. It was as if Mom slashed me with the knife she was holding. I was terribly disappointed. I did not say anything, but I took my essay and went to my room. From then on I hated my brother. I had no guilt feelings and I was aware that I wished he would die."

His relations with his parents deteriorated. He concentrated on his studies. He chose to go to college two thousand miles away, and he tried to avoid visiting his parents whenever possible. His relations with women were casual, and, generally speaking, he was not particularly attached to anyone. When the evaluator inquired about these monastic tendencies of his, he smiled bitterly and answered somewhat irrelevantly. "What's the use?" he said, "I don't care about art anymore. I majored in chemistry." The following exchange then took place:

EVALUATOR: Are you willing to revive your interest in art?

PATIENT: I don't think that I would be here if I didn't.

EVALUATOR: It seems to me that your isolation, in general, and from women, in particular, has to do with this rejection that you experienced from your mother. Do you think that if we focused our attention during the next few months on disentangling your feelings for your mother that this would be a good area to concentrate on and try to solve?

PATIENT: Yes, I think so, because I assure you that I'm tired of this isolation. Deep inside I know that I like people.

EVALUATOR: I'm sure you do.

To summarize what has been said up to now about the Oedipal focus, there appear to be three categories of Oedipal problem. The first category includes those patients who linger a bit too long in their attachment to the parent of the opposite sex, tending to procrastinate in choosing to abandon their wishes for and competition with their parents and in finding a suitable surrogate among their peers. These patients, of course, are the best STAPP candidates, and invariably they are able to overcome their difficulties without much difficulty.

The second category provides a somewhat more complex picture and includes those patients who in one way or another were encouraged by their parents to remain attached to them. Examples might be when a father clearly prefers his daughter over his other children and thus acts seductively toward her. Another example would be the father who, because of his work or other reasons, is frequently absent, thus leaving his son and wife together over long periods of time. If the mother has a preference for her son, she may encourage his remaining attached to her. Thus a father and mother who manage by their behavior to support their children's attachment to them tend to make it more difficult for their children to become independent.

Finally, the third category presents the most complications. Here a major external event in the form of a realistic life situation occurring during the Oedipal period tends to create difficulties that cannot be changed and presents the patient with certain problems that appear at face value almost insurmountable. They clearly interfere with the resolution of his Oedipus complex. These have to do with such things as the death or the permanent separation of the parents. Thus, if one parent is eliminated and if this is the parent with whom the patient is competing, he feels victorious in this struggle. Despite the guilt feelings which are likely to be aroused during such circumstances, the patient is tempted to remain attached to the parent of the opposite sex and is reluctant to proceed with the search for a parental substitute. Patients who fall into this last category tend to have the greatest difficulty with the resolution of their Oedipal problem and are the most difficult of all our candidates to treat.

Before we leave the subject of the establishment of an Oedipal focus as a prerequisite for STAPP, if not for other kinds of brief dynamic psychotherapy, I can state categorically that from our experience, contrary to certain prevailing theoretic considerations, a true resolution of the Oedipus complex in women is possible just as it is in men. We are, therefore, in agreement with Gray's (1976) theoretical discussion and conclusions about this subject, and we think that suitable female patients are just as good candidates for STAPP as their male counterparts may be.

Thus in STAPP we deal with Oedipal problems in which *positive feelings* for both parents predominate and conflicts do arise when the patient is forced to make a choice. In patients whose negative feelings seem to predominate as a result of what they might, for example, interpret as a rejection by the parent of the opposite sex, whether or not they feel competition with the parent of the same sex, the difficulties which are likely to be encountered are much more complex. As a result, it is possible that their treatment would have to be prolonged. Similar difficulties may also appear to be the result of psychopathology not only in the patient but also in one or both of his parents.

Finally, it should not be forgotten that the Oedipus complex is the nuclear complex and represents the essential part in the content of neuroses; thus it is an appropriate focus on which to concentrate during psychotherapy.

We are now ready to deal with the final evaluation task, the "therapeutic contract."

THE "THERAPEUTIC CONTRACT"

The "therapeutic contract" constitutes a mutual agreement about the therapeutic focus on which the treatment is to be based.

It is up to the evaluator, therefore, to summarize succinctly his impression of the patient's problem based on the information obtained during the history taking. He must also be able to substantiate this impression by solid evidence in the form of specific examples of events, fantasies, and memories given to him by the patient and amassed during the course of the whole evaluation.

This presentation by the evaluator must be agreed upon by the patient, and thus the "therapeutic contract" establishes clearly the limits of their future therapeutic work. In addition, it lays the foundation for the development of a therapeutic alliance which cements the two participants of the dyadic relationship, and which, at difficult times in the course of therapy, acts as a motivating force to help the patient overcome his problems and arrive at a meaningful solution.

This is not to imply, however, that the evaluator always knows best or is always right. By virtue of his lack of emotional investment in the patient's difficulties, his ability to be objective, and his professional knowledge and experience, the evaluator is in a good position to outline the therapeutic focus. He should be cautious, however, not to jump to quick conclusions. If, for example, the patient hesitates to accept his formulation and is unsure about the focus, the evaluator should investigate further the sources of this resistance and must be willing to change the emphasis of the therapeutic focus if this appears justified.

It is obvious from all that has already been said that one of the most interesting aspects of short-term psychotherapeutic work has to do with the infinitesimal variations in pattern and style which we encounter in our daily interactions with our patients and with our ability to choose the important factors on which to concentrate. Since no two patients are exactly the same, no two therapeutic formulations can be equated; despite all similarities, one should not impose the same therapeutic focus on one patient because it has worked out well on another patient with a similar problem. Thus the evaluator should be careful to tailor-make a therapeutic focus for each individual patient.

The ease with which a patient agrees with the evaluation, on the other hand, may imply a degree of passivity on his part which should be considered with suspicion.

Looking back at our therapeutic failures, I am convinced that the majority were due to a faulty evaluation of certain pregenital character traits which pointed to the existence of a more serious psychopathology. The three most important of these are passivity, excessive dependence, and "acting-out" or manipulative tendencies.

At face value, it should be fairly easy to evaluate basic defects in these pregenital characterological areas, and with most patients this is indeed the case. Occasionally, however, problems arise when the evaluator is misled or underestimates the importance of seemingly mild passive, dependent, or acting-out personality traits. Here is an example:

A 28-year-old Ph.D. candidate complained that for about a year she had wished to withdraw from people. Although she mentioned that at other times during her life she had detected similar wishes, she felt that at the present time these wishes were very intense. She related that, during the previous summer, she had taken a job in a laboratory, doing some work on her thesis, and had become involved with another doctoral candidate named Jack, whose work she admired greatly and to whom she had felt sexually attracted. Unfortunately, the relationship did not develop according to her expectations; she soon started to feel mildly depressed and developed a desire to be alone, away from people. Her work did not suffer, however, and she was able almost to finish her dissertation.

Her father was a scientist, and she had always been attached to him. She was able to give many good examples of the closeness of their relationship while she was quite young, but during her early adolescence her father's behavior became erratic following a severe illness, and at times he would disappear for weeks without anyone knowing where he was. Her relations with her mother and her older sister were good, and she indicated that, whenever she visited them, she had such a good time that she did not want to leave.

The patient seemed to fulfill the selection of criteria, and the therapeutic focus was considered to be an Oedipal one involving a repetition of her attachment to her father, as well as traumatic separations from him, in her relationships with other men. The female evaluator communicated this to the patient, who readily agreed with her impression and was willing to work in this area of her interpersonal difficulties. During the clinic intake conference the patient was also interviewed by a male psychiatrist who was in general agreement with this previously outlined therapeutic focus. He did feel, however, that the patient did not relate to him as well as she had been described as relating to the female evaluator. He also observed that the patient seemed to procrastinate a little toward the end of the interview, indicating a desire to prolong it. Nevertheless, the patient was accepted for STAPP and was assigned to a female therapist.

As soon as therapy started, the nature of her dependent needs appeared and, although the therapist tried to bypass them (a technical requirement for STAPP which will be discussed later in detail), she seemed to be unsuccessful. For example, the patient demanded to be seen twice a week when she found out that her therapist was going away on a two-week vacation and became teary when the therapist refused her request. Following her return, the therapist found the patient depressed. Her interest in men had vanished and she seemed to have regressed. The therapist was unable despite her efforts to return to the agreed-upon focus and had difficulty satisfying the patient's dependent needs.

What went wrong? Nothing more, than that greater attention should have been paid to the patient's enjoyment of relationships with women and her pseudoheterosexual interests. It was our underestimation of the extent and depth of the patient's dependent needs that led to the failure of STAPP in a patient who, in other respects, appeared to be a good candidate for this kind of treatment.

Another factor which in my opinion also contributed to this failure had to do with one of the patient's statements during the discussion of the "therapeutic contract." Although the patient readily agreed with the therapeutic focus outlined by the evaluator, she added: "Of course, there's another problem which may be connected with my tendency to want to withdraw from people, which is clearly associated with my past experiences with my father. This has to do with my need to cling to Jack although I know he doesn't love me." The evaluator was noncommittal on this point but emphasized that she thought the patient's problem was primarily related to the difficulties with her father. The patient agreed with this, and the subject of "clinging to Jack," instead of being further clarified, was dropped. Although pregenital characterological issues are avoided during the course of STAPP because the therapist is reasonably certain that they are of minor importance, they should be investigated very extensively during the evaluation process if they are, at face value, not severe.

Finally, the therapeutic contract serves the purpose of making the patient take an active responsibility in the development of his psychotherapeutic work and sharing the difficulty which will be encountered as an *equal* partner, not as one dependent on the evaluator.

There is one task left for the evaluator to perform which, although it may not be an integral part of the evaluation process, makes a valuable contribution to the assessment of the therapeutic outcome. This task is referred to as "the specification of criteria for successful therapeutic results."

Having had the opportunity to assess the patient's psychological problem, the evaluator should be able to state, preferably in writing, what in his opinion will constitute a resolution of this specific patient's idiosyncratic difficulties, both psychodynamically and phenomenologically. Thus he should specify, for example, whether the symptoms will be eliminated, in what way the interpersonal difficulties would change, and with what members of the patient's family circle. He should make a prediction about changes in the patient's self-esteem and self-understanding. The ability to learn new ways to handle his emotional conflicts should be mentioned, with notations made about the substitution of more adaptive defense mechanisms for those which are maladaptive. Some statements should be made about the patient's future capability to solve his psychological problems, giving specific examples of not only having adhered to this goal but also of utilizing this newly acquired problem-solving ability in his future life. These specifications made at the end of the evaluation should be tested by independent evaluation at the end of the therapy in order to see whether or not the predictions have been fulfilled. The concept of specifying outcome criteria before and after short-term psychotherapy is one of the most valuable contributions to psychotherapy research, and we are indebted to Malan (1976c), who was the first to formulate it.

The following questionnaire, which is now used routinely by all the evaluators in the psychiatric clinic of the Beth Israel Hospital, and which has also been used at the Psykiatrisk Klinikk of the University of Oslo, Norway, attempts to synthesize all that I have been discussing in the last three chapters. It has proven to be of invaluable assistance in surveying our patient population and in selecting appropriate patients to receive the kind of treatment best suited to their needs.

CRITERIA FOR SELECTION OF PATIENTS

Patient's Name _____ Evaluation No._____
Address_____
_____
Interviewer _____ Date _____
Type of Interview: ___ Evaluation   ___ Administrative   ___ Research
Please check *Yes* or *No* on each question. Do not check both or put a question mark in the middle.

Part A   Yes   No

1. Can the patient circumscribe his/her chief complaint or assign top priority to one out of several difficulties? (The above question should be answered after the evaluator has helped the patient define his/her chief complaint.)   ___   ___
    a. Is the chief complaint a symptom? If so, please underline: anxiety, depression, obsession, compulsion, conversion, phobia, other_____   ___   ___
    b. Is the chief complaint a problem in interpersonal relations? If so, with whom? Please specify _____   ___   ___
2. As a result of systematic history taking can you identify at least *one meaningful relationship* in the patient's childhood? (This implies an ability on the part of the patient to make a sacrifice for another person, or to give up a part of his/her pleasure for a loved one. Meaningful means "give-and-take, altruistic" relationship.)   ___   ___
3. Can the patient interact flexibly with the evaluator by expressing feelings appropriately during the interview?   ___   ___
4. Is the patient psychologically minded? (This question attempts to assess the patient's psychological sophistication as well as a general level of above-average intelligence. In answering this question, please keep in mind both of the above factors. Excellence in work or educational performance should be helpful factors in answering this question.)   ___   ___
5. Does the patient show adequate motivation for *change?* (This does not imply a motivation for symptom relief or for psychotherapy. The patient must be tired of his/her problems, and be willing to make an effort to alter his/her neurotic behavior.)   ___   ___
    a. Can the patient recognize that the symptoms are psychological in origin?   ___   ___
    b. Is the patient honest in reporting about himself?   ___   ___
    c. Is the patient willing to participate actively in the evaluation?   ___   ___
    d. Is the patient introspective, and actively curious about himself?   ___   ___
    e. Does the patient really desire to change and not simply to have the symptoms removed?   ___   ___

Yes   No

   f. Are the expectations of the results of the treatment *realistic* (i.e., not grandiose, magical, etc.)?   —   —

   g. Is the patient willing to make a reasonable and tangible sacrifice (e.g., see the therapist at a mutually convenient time, pay a reasonable fee)?   —   —

Part B

6. Is there an *Oedipal problem* (triangular, genital heterosexual) which has been clearly established during the evaluation, can explain primarily the patient's psychodynamics, can become the focus for the psychotherapy, and if resolved can eliminate the patient's difficulties?   —   —

7. If your answer to question 6 is no, please specify if in your opinion there is another focus on which the psychotherapy could concentrate, such as loss of a loved one or another.—

_____

_____

Part C

8. Please predict all specific changes that will constitute a successful therapeutic outcome for this individual patient. (For example: absence of phobia, depression, etc.; improved relations with wife; no need to depend on father or mother to support patient; improved relations with boss, boyfriend, daughter, etc.; better work or educational performance; better relations with men or women.) *Please specify several criteria.*

_____

_____

_____

_____

_____

9. Please indicate your recommended therapy by underlining one of the following: (a) STAPP; (b) brief psychotherapy (other kinds); (c) long-term dynamic psychotherapy; (d) brief supportive psychotherapy; (e) long-term supportive psychotherapy; (f) supportive psychotherapy with medication; (g) behavior modification; (h) group therapy; (i) hypnotherapy; (j) crisis support; (k) crisis intervention; (l) couples therapy; (m) relaxation techniques; (n) other:_____

Part D

Does the patient:

10. a. show adequate self-esteem?   —   —
    b. have potential to show adequate self-esteem?   —   —

11. a. have the ability to solve his/her emotional problem?   —   —
    b. have the potential to solve his/her emotional problem?   —   —

12. a. have the ability to understand himself/herself?   —   —
    b. have the potential to understand himself/herself?   —   —

13. Is the patient in a state of emotional crisis?   —   —

14. Is he/she under the influence of external stress?   —   —

Part E

15. Is the patient able to form a therapeutic alliance?   —   —

	Yes	No
16. Do you like the patient?	—	—
17. Will the patient's symptoms improve?	—	—
18. Will the patient's interpersonal relations improve?	—	—
19. Do you predict that therapy will be successful?	—	—

20. Please rank your overall impression of the patient as a can-
    didate for STAPP on a scale from 0 to 100 _____
                        (0 = bad;   100 = good)

Part F

Diagnosis _____
_____

PART TWO

TECHNIQUE

CHAPTER 5

The Opening Phase of STAPP

In my book *Short-Term Psychotherapy and Emotional Crisis* (Sifneos, 1972) I discussed at some length the specific requirements for STAPP. To avoid repetition, therefore, I shall only summarize the major points here.

REQUIREMENTS

The interviews are held once a week, at a specified time. The patient must understand that the therapist will keep the appointed time open for him and he must therefore feel responsible for keeping his appointment. He should be prepared to discuss any planned alterations or cancellations in advance and to pay for any missed interviews. These somewhat strict requirements are aimed at giving the patient the impression that the therapist takes his therapeutic role very seriously and assigns a high priority to it.

It is best that the appointments be made at a specified time. Although it may be mutually convenient for the patient as well as for the therapist to change the day or the time of the interview, this should be avoided unless it is absolutely necessary. Such changes give the patient an opportunity to act out, yet it is more difficult for the therapist to deal with such an acting-out when it may be par tially related to realistic factors. For example, a patient used the traffic as an excuse for being late. Once it was the morning traffic; the next time it was the afternoon traffic. These excuses were partially true but were also associated with a resistance on his part to talk about a need to compete and have a contest with men, in general, as well as with the therapist. Since the appointments kept being switched by the therapist because of his own schedule, the patient was able to continue acting-out. When the therapist finally dealt with this issue of the traffic, the patient switched his tactics and started having problems with finding a parking space.

Of course, such difficulties may also occur when the appointment is at a specified time, but then the therapist knows exactly what the traffic or parking conditions are at that time and can deal quickly with any acting-out tendency appropriately and early.

The length of the interview is 45 minutes, and the time cannot be prolonged beyond that limit. This is done to discourage those patients who tend to cling to their therapists and want to extend the length of their interview, as well as those who bring up what they consider to be an important subject during the last few minutes of the interview to create a situation in which they can compete or manipulate the therapist in an effort to control him.

Although STAPP is a psychodynamic psychotherapy based on theoretical psychoanalytic principles, the interviews are held face to face, and the patient is not asked either to lie on a couch looking away from the therapist or to free-associate. Since the emphasis in STAPP is a focalization, all the factors, environmental or otherwise, which can be helpful to achieve this task are used as extensively as possible.

The face-to-face interviews tend to discourage the ramblings which many patients use to avoid facing some unpleasant truths about themselves following an anxiety-provoking confrontation by their therapists. After these points have been clarified, both participants should be ready to embark on the serious problem-solving venture of STAPP.

LIMITATION OF TIME

There are some differences of opinion about what is meant by time limitation in short-term dynamic therapy. On the one hand,

Mann (1973) has developed a therapy which he calls "time limited" and which requires only 12 interviews for all his patients. Others, such as Strupp and his colleagues, limit the therapy to 25 to 30 hours (Strupp, 1984). Malan sets up a termination date at the time of the evaluation. His brief therapy usually lasts between 30 and 40 sessions. Davanloo, Gillieron, Guyotat, and Brusset, in Montreal, Lausanne, Lyon, and Paris, respectively, also set up a termination date but appear to be fairly flexible about it (Brusset, 1983; Davanloo, 1980; Gillieron, 1983; Buyotat, 1983).

In STAPP we leave the termination of the treatment open-ended. We think that every patient should be allowed to resolve the psychological problem which they have agreed to investigate at their own pace, but over a short period of time. Usually STAPP patients achieve a resolution of their difficulties in a two- to six-month period.

There was only one patient whose treatment lasted just under one year. During his evaluation it was decided that he was an excellent candidate for STAPP, fulfilling all the criteria and having an unresolved Oedipal focus. When I assigned the patient to one of our PGY-5 residents who had a great deal of experience in long-term psychotherapy but who also wanted to learn STAPP, he asked me whether he could be supervised by one of his current supervisors, who also was interested in STAPP. I agreed reluctantly. The therapy went on for about four months. When I asked the resident how things were going, he told me that everything was proceeding smoothly. After six months went by, I became apprehensive, thinking that we might have picked up the wrong STAPP patient, but the resident assured me that all was going along fine. At nine months I became panicky. When I asked the therapist what was going wrong, he told me that he and his supervisor were working on the patient's feelings about his grandfather's death. Exasperated, I pointed out to him that he should have been working on the unresolved Oedipal focus and not offering long-term therapy to the patient. He was finally able to help the patient resolve his Oedipal feelings, and the therapy came to an end after lasting almost one year.

I saw the patient as an independent evaluator after his treatment was over and I was satisfied that he had been able to resolve his Oedipal competition successfully. When I asked him how he liked his therapist, he went on as follows:

PATIENT: I really liked Dr. N very much. He was very sensitive and
  he helped me to understand my problem, but (*hesitating*)—I have
  one question in my mind.
EVALUATOR: And what was that?
PATIENT: I don't know why he was so much interested in my grandfather's death!

I learned my lesson. From then on Dr. Fishman—a member of
our research team—and I supervised all STAPP with our residents.

All short-term dynamic psychotherapies are based on psychoanalytic principles, but the technical issues used by various workers
in the field may vary considerably.

Here is a list of the technical issues used in STAPP. They will
be discussed in greater detail in the following chapters.

1. Consolidations of the working alliance and its transforma-
   tions into a therapeutic alliance
2. Early utilization of positive transference feelings
3. Countertransference issues
4. Sex of the therapist
5. Activity of the therapist
6. Focality during the course of the therapy
7. Use of anxiety-provoking questions, confrontations, and
   clarifications
8. Therapist—parent connections or past-transference link
   interpretations
9. Avoidance of pregenital characterological issues used by the
   patient defensively, and of development of a transference
   neurosis
10. New learning and problem solving
11. Short-term predictions between sessions and note taking
12. Recapitulation at times of massive resistance
13. Support of patient who is making progress
14. Education of the patient
15. Tangible evidence of change and development of insight
16. Early termination

THE FIRST INTERVIEW

The opening statements of the patient in STAPP, as in psychoanalysis, at times contain a communication which represents in

summary form all the main aspects of the patient's psychological problem. The patient should therefore be encouraged to begin his therapy by talking about any subject of his own choosing. There are patients, on the other hand, who deliberately prefer to be vague because they have sensed that the focalization is going to make them anxious. Here is an example:

A 25-year-old social worker expressed concern because she claimed to have forgotten what the area of concentration for her therapy was going to be. She went on as follows:

PATIENT: I know that it may be significant, but the funny thing about it is that I cannot remember what we agreed to talk about last week.

THERAPIST: Why is it funny?

PATIENT: I meant it in the sense that it was peculiar.

THERAPIST: But you used the word "funny." What's so amusing in forgetting what we decided to focus on during your therapy?

PATIENT: Well, it must have something to do with wanting some guidance of sorts. If I don't remember, then you will help me.

THERAPIST: Yet, how can I help you when I don't know as yet why you have the problems that bring you to the clinic.

PATIENT: That's true.

THERAPIST: So, there is a part of you which nevertheless wants me to do something which you know only too well I cannot do. Now, assuming that I tried to tell you what to talk about, how would you feel about it?

PATIENT: I'd like it.

THERAPIST: Part of you would like it, but how would the other part feel? The part that knows that I cannot do it?

PATIENT: A little silly.

THERAPIST: Meaning . . .

PATIENT (hesitating):—That you are a little silly, doing something like that when you really don't know.

THERAPIST: Precisely! So, wouldn't it be funny, then, to see your therapist do something silly?

PATIENT: In a way, yes.

THERAPIST: So the word "funny" was used appropriately.

PATIENT: I suppose so.

THERAPIST: Now that we have clarified this point, let's return to your lapse of memory.

PATIENT: The funny thing is that I have just remembered what we have agreed to concentrate on during my treatment.

THERAPIST: There are a lot of funny things going on today! Why don't you carry on?

As must be obvious to the reader, the therapy with this patient starts immediately on a transference issue. What is striking, however, is the patient's willingness to understand and cooperate with the therapist's attempt to clarify the situation.

Here is an example of the opening phase of STAPP with a patient who continues to think about the therapeutic focus which was agreed upon and brings up associations which are pertinent and promote self-understanding. A 21-year-old female college senior started her first interview as follows:

PATIENT: I have been thinking about what you and I discussed at the end of our interview last week and I had a memory which popped into mind that I had not thought of for a long time. Shall I tell you about it, or is there something else that I'm supposed to be talking about?

There are several responses available to the therapist in his reaction to this opening statement. He may simply express interest and encourage the patient to provide more information or he may choose to instruct the patient as to what indeed is expected to take place during the psychotherapeutic interview. Another approach would be to avoid showing interest in the specific memory, which the patient may use as a bait in order to manipulate the therapist by arousing his interest. In that case, he may choose to ask in return some questions not directly related to the specific memory. Finally, since the patient is referring to certain expectations she may have about the role of the therapist, he may respond as follows:

THERAPIST: You seem to think that I have certain expectations of the specific issues that you are supposed to be talking about. Can you tell me something more about this?

It is obvious that each therapist would judge what is the most appropriate response to the opening remarks of the patient. In this case, the therapist was impressed by the patient's motivation to understand herself and decided that it was important to hear about what she had remembered during the previous week. He chose, therefore, to respond as follows, trying to deal with as many of these factors as possible:

THERAPIST: There is no rule as to what you should or what you should not talk about. You are just as good a judge of what is important and what is not as I am. It's obvious, however, that you have some expectation that I should guide you. If you have any more thoughts about this, please talk about them, because what goes on between the two of us is important and must be understood. Now, you mentioned this episode that popped into your mind during the past week. Which one of all these things do you want to talk about?

PATIENT: I see! So you want me to be the judge. Okay, I like that. Well! You remember last time that you asked me about special interactions that I may have had with my father when I was young. I kept thinking about your question after I left the office. I had told you about my father's always helping me with my math. He did seem, however, to be a bit impatient, particularly when he was reading a book or his newspaper, but he would do it nevertheless. What occurred to me as I left was that I was perfectly capable of doing all my math alone and of solving the problems without his help. I was a very good student and I didn't need any assistance. So the question was, why did I have to run to my father? The obvious answer to it was that I wanted to get his attention and to distract him from what he was doing in order to engage him in some activity with me.

THERAPIST: And what was this memory which you remembered? (*Satisfied that the patient is indeed working hard to resolve her problem by actively thinking about the focal issue of her relationship with her father, the therapist somewhat impatiently asks for information about what in his opinion seems to be an important recollection.*)

PATIENT: It was on a Sunday. My father was reading his thick newspaper, drinking his beer, and looking very relaxed. My youngest brother was playing with his cars, racing them around my father's chair. My father suddenly stopped reading, put the paper down, and, looking fascinated, watched my brother's games with his little cars. Soon after, he asked my brother how was he able to make the cars race around so fast and he started to laugh when my brother showed him how he was doing it. At that point I started to feel irritated. I knew that Bob—that was my brother's name—was my father's favorite because he was the youngest. . . . (*The patient was silent for a while.*)

THERAPIST (*interrupting her silence*): What are you thinking about right now?

PATIENT: Oh, I had an irrelevant thought! It occurred to me that my father never played with my dolls when I was Bob's age. So at that point I went to my father and said, "Daddy, I have a difficult algebra problem. Can you help me out? We have a quiz tomorrow." My father got up, told Bob that he had to work with me on my math, because it was more important than racing with the little cars. Bob looked sad but continued to play. My father and I went to the study to do my algebra. (*The patient was silent again.*)

THERAPIST: Is that all?

PATIENT: Well, almost.

THERAPIST: What more was there?

PATIENT (*blushing*): I must admit something that I don't like and really that is what I remembered primarily during this week. It was that I invented the whole thing. You see, it was all a lie I told my father. There was no quiz the next day. I just lied. . . .

THERAPIST: Because you were jealous?

PATIENT: Yes, because I was jealous.

This type of reaction during the first interview is quite typical of many STAPP patients. Their curiosity having been aroused by the material that has been discussed during the therapy session, they are motivated to examine their reactions, to look into themselves, and to add to their self-understanding. Although the beginning of a working alliance has already begun to develop during the evaluation, it is important that the therapist try to cement it further by stressing the joint and collaborative nature of their therapeutic task. Thus, the working alliance between the therapist and the patient must now evolve into a true therapeutic alliance.

THE THERAPEUTIC ALLIANCE

The establishment of a therapeutic alliance is one of the best technical dimensions of STAPP. In the example which I have discussed, the therapist had the therapeutic alliance in mind when he commented to the patient that she was just as good a judge of what was important to be talked about as he was. He was clearly implying that they had to work together and that the patient's contributions were just as important as, or even more important than, his own. Here is another example:

A 24-year-old male graduate student described difficulties in his interpersonal relations with both men and women as follows:

PATIENT: I put on an act. I wear a mask. I give the impression that I'm different from what I really am. I don't like this attitude in me.

THERAPIST: Can you give me an example?

PATIENT: What happened last week is a case in point. Before my girlfriend broke off our relationship, she said that she didn't like going out with someone who is "a phony." She said that she didn't really think that I was one but that she was tired of seeing me putting on an act. Mary, my previous girlfriend, had said the same thing, using different words, and so did Bob, my best friend. I know what they are all talking about. At times, even here, I have this great urge to show off to make you admire me. I succeed up to a certain point on the outside. But eventually I overdo it, obviously, and these people see through my act, and then they get tired of all this show.

THERAPIST: And where does this urge come from?

PATIENT: From very long ago. I used to put on an act to impress my mother. I remember one time when I made up a whole story about school. I told her that the teacher had said I was the best student she had ever had. My mother was impressed, but you know, doctor, it wasn't true. The teacher had complimented me, but I exaggerated it. I blew it out of proportion.

THERAPIST: So you were trying to impress your mother, you are trying to impress your girlfriends, and Bob, and even here—

PATIENT: What do you mean "even here"?

THERAPIST: A minute ago you said that even here you had such a tendency.

PATIENT: Did I say that?

THERAPIST: Yes, you did. Furthermore, why does it surprise you? If you put on an act with everyone else, why wouldn't you put on an act with me?

PATIENT: It did occur to me that it was possible, but this is precisely what I don't want to do. I'm here to understand why I do it so I can stop pretending. I want you to help me.

THERAPIST: Of course. I appreciate your motivation and I'll try to help you, but the first thing that we can expect is that there will be another part of you with the urge to put on a facade to cover up. We should be prepared to face this and to see where this tendency originates, what its purpose is, and what it achieves for you.

PATIENT: Yes, that's exactly what I want to do.

Despite the potential for deception on the part of the patient within the therapeutic situation, it is clear that his motivation to understand himself is strong. The therapist takes advantage of it early in the therapy to strengthen the therapeutic alliance. Later in the same interview the following exchange took place:

THERAPIST: We have already seen that these tendencies of yours had something to do with your mother. Can you tell me something more about this?

PATIENT: Yes, I know it's true, but what else is there to say?

THERAPIST: Can you be more specific? Can you give me an example?

PATIENT: I can't think of anything right now. . . .

THERAPIST: I did not mean necessarily to ask for more general information but rather for a more specific example from the past, so that we can try to tie together the present experiences with those that occurred in your childhood.

PATIENT: I thought it was your job to tie all these things together.

THERAPIST: No, not exactly. It is not an "either/or" or "your task or mine," but rather a joint venture. You know, in the final analysis it is your ability to learn to solve your own problems that counts, isn't it?

PATIENT: Yes, I agree . . . okay, let me think. Well, one thing that occurs to me is about school. I remember that I disliked baseball and I didn't want to stay at school and play ball with the other kids after class, so I would invent some excuse to tell the teacher that I had to go home. Now, the real reason was that I wanted to be home with my mother, but I couldn't tell that to the teacher. She would have thought that I was a sissy, a mama's boy, so I invented a story.

THERAPIST: But was this done only for the teacher, or could it be that it served some other purpose?

PATIENT: . . . What do you mean?

THERAPIST: What comes to mind in reference to my question?

PATIENT: I don't know what you really want, what you're aiming at.

THERAPIST: I want nothing.

PATIENT: Yes, I know. It's both of us . . . let me see, then. Well, my father comes to mind.

THERAPIST: In what way?

PATIENT: My father was a traveling salesman, as I told you, but I remember that at times he would come back unexpectedly. One day when I was at home, having skipped class, I was talking with my mother when my dad walked in on us. He was surprised to see me home and asked me what I was doing. I blurted out that I had a sore throat, which wasn't true. My father was very sympathetic about it and I felt guilty for lying to him.

THERAPIST: So, lying had a double purpose, to fool both the teacher and your father. It kept both of them in the dark about your real intentions. We know now that the real reason was to be home with your mother.

PATIENT: Yes, it's true.

From this exchange it is clear that the therapist has already achieved the cooperation of the patient, and meaningful information is already flowing out. By asking the patient to be more specific, the therapist not only discourages the use of vague generalizations but also emphasizes that only specific, tangible examples will help their work. Furthermore he gives a strong and clear message to the patient about the nature of their cooperation. It is evident, in this case, that the therapeutic alliance has already been forged by the end of the first interview.

There are also didactic elements in the therapist's attitude when he prepares the patient as to what to expect during the treatment and, in some way, when he sets down the rules which are to be followed. There is a similarity here with the analyst who instructs the analysand about the basic rules of psychoanalysis. This didactic task helps to make an even transition from the ending of the evaluation to the beginning of STAPP.

In reference to this transition, however, I should emphasize that there is no clear-cut line of demarcation between the end of the evaluation and the beginning of therapy. Both processes overlap, of course, but I find it easier to keep them in mind clearly as two distinct entities so as to develop a conceptual frame of reference for any discussion of the evaluation process and the early therapy.

Because of this, I find it helpful to announce to the patient when the evaluation has come to an end. I do this by summarizing my impressions of the problem to be solved and by recapitulating the therapeutic focus on which the therapy will revolve and which has already been discussed in detail. It is like giving a signal for the therapy to start.

THE THERAPEUTIC VALUE OF A SINGLE INTERVIEW

At times, however, the therapeutic impact of the evaluation or of the first interview is such that there is no need for further psychotherapy because in reality the patient's problem is actually being solved. Here are two examples from our clinic population, one with a male and another with a female patient:

A 29-year-old junior executive complained that his marriage was on the verge of collapse because his wife had had an affair with her boss, who was also a good friend of his. He related that he was surprised by his reaction of rage at his friend while feeling little, if any, anger at his wife, who in his opinion had actually seduced his friend.

He was the second of three boys. He came from a wealthy family and was very much attached to his mother, although he believed that she preferred his older brother. As he was talking about his mother, he remembered an episode from his youth, when she was reading him a story before putting him to bed. It appears that the patient suggested that his mother stop and urged her instead to read the story to his brother, who was sick and who had not gone to school. He remembered that his mother had been impressed by his altruism and complimented him on his spirit of self-sacrifice. Having accepted his suggestion, however, she left him, and he recalled crying bitterly when he heard her voice coming from his brother's room.

As he grew older, he thought he had accepted his mother's

subtle favoritism toward his older brother. He attributed this to his brother's being thin and dark, taking after her side of the family, whereas the patient resembled his father. His relations with his brothers were described as stormy. They fought a great deal, and on occasion, using his greater weight, he was able to push his brother around although he was three years his junior. He felt very proud during these occasions.

During college he got much better grades than his brother and graduated with honors from business school, whereas his brother had decided against going to graduate school. The relation with his younger brother, 10 years his junior, was uneventful. He also described his father, who was a successful banker, as aloof and distant. The patient had met and soon married his wife three years before coming to seek psychiatric help. He described her as being tall, ash blonde, somewhat on the heavy side, with pale-blue eyes. Their difficulties seemed to have started soon after their wedding, when he tried to convince her that she should be independent and urged her to get a job. Despite her initial reluctance she acquiesced, but their quarreling continued, particularly when he pressed her to attend evening business meetings and when he gave her long lectures about how to succeed in the business world, which she resented. On one occasion he told his wife that she should accept her boss's offer to accompany him on a trip to the West Coast, despite her objections. "I know Bill," he told his wife. "He gets very lonely when he travels and is prone to making serious errors of judgment. He needs someone to watch over him."

At this point the therapist felt that a tentative confrontation was in order so as to observe the patient's reaction to it. He went on as follows:

THERAPIST: You mean to say that you urged your wife to go on that business trip in the same way as you told your mother to go and read the story to your brother?

PATIENT (*silent and reflecting*): . . . . I never thought of these two episodes in this context . . . hm. . . .

THERAPIST: So, then, we may say that you view your wife in the same way as you viewed your mother when you were younger?

PATIENT: Yes, this is true. Come to think of it, I seem to have had the same feeling, the same urge, the same need to convince them to do what I recommended. On the other hand, there's a great deal of difference between my mother and Mary, because they look so different. Mother is thin and dark.

THERAPIST: They do look different, but they share the same name. They are both called Mrs. R.

PATIENT: Wow! (*He was quiet for a while and then, looking very sad, he went on*): I had such a good time with Mary before we were married. Something happened afterward. I was vaguely aware of it. . . .

THERAPIST: Now we do know what happened. Mary changed her name and she became instantly like your mother. She also received all the feelings of jealousy which you had for your mother and brother which you displaced on her, and you managed to send her into the arms of her boss.

PATIENT: It's amazing how the mind works!

In the beginning of the following interview, the patient said that he did not think that he needed any more psychotherapy. His therapist was surprised by this and thought, at first, that he was fleeing from his treatment because of the anxiety-provoking confrontations of the first session, but when questioned about his reasons for wanting to stop, the patient said:

PATIENT: I have done a lot of thinking after my last hour here. When I left your office, all kinds of memories came to my mind which confirmed what we discovered in here. It was clear that I had displaced my feelings for my mother onto poor Mary. What clinched it was the realization that I had not been angry at my wife when she told me about having an affair with her boss, but that I felt furious at him in the same way as I had felt angry and jealous at my brother Joe, and I was so happy when I could push him around physically. I had actually thought of going to the office and beating Bill up. Can you imagine that? A civilized human being like me entertaining such thoughts! I felt guilty and ashamed. It was all exactly alike. Three days ago I talked with Mary and I apologized to her for my behavior. I also asked her to reconsider her decision to get a divorce. I admitted that I had made many mistakes. She was not very sympathetic and I don't blame her. I am hopeful, however, because I think that deep inside my wife still loves me and she doesn't want a divorce. I actually detected some changes in her attitude toward me the last few days. She seems more friendly somehow. In any case, whatever happens, it doesn't matter. I do understand things much better now. That interview here last week was very important. I don't like to be melodramatic, but it made a great impact on my life.

These words speak for themselves.

Here is what happened in the first interview of a 24-year-old female receptionist who came to the clinic complaining of feeling depressed because she fought constantly with her stepfather, and because these fights made her life miserable. She added that her mother was also very disturbed by what was going on and that her stepfather, who at face value pretended to show little emotion and put on a calm exterior, was actually also quite unhappy. She said that the difficulties with her stepfather had lasted more than 10 years. Although she had thought of moving out of her parents' house, she found excuses not to do so.

She was born in Ireland. Her father died when she was four, and her mother came to the United States. She indicated that she had had a happy childhood. She had considered herself as being her parents' favorite because she was the youngest of four children and because she was the only girl. The difficulties with her stepfather, who married her mother when the patient was twelve years old, had started after an episode which she seemed embarrassed to talk about. It appears that her mother had been hospitalized and that everyone was quite worried about an operation which was scheduled for the following day. She remembered that her stepfather had had several drinks before dinner, which surprised her because he usually drank very little. She had gone to bed early, having to go to some kind of school activity early the following day. She was suddenly awakened during the night and found her stepfather sitting on her bed and caressing her breasts. The patient was embarrassed. She pushed him away and he staggered away swearing. She said that she felt very upset following this episode but was willing to forget it, attributing her stepfather's behavior to his being upset about her mother's operation. She also said that she felt sorry for him. It was her stepfather, however, who changed completely soon afterward. Instead of being friendly and loving, he became very irritable and seemed to go out of his way to find fault with her and to criticize her. She was very upset by this turn of events and could not understand why it was happening.

THERAPIST: Has it occurred to you that your stepfather had to be angry with you so as to protect himself from repeating the scene at your bed?

PATIENT (*flabbergasted*): I never thought of it that way . . . (*She was silent for a while and then she added*): That puts a very different emphasis on the whole thing, doesn't it?

The therapist agreed and asked her to talk about her relations with men in general. She said that she had only casual acquaintances during high school and college, but that the last two summers she had traveled in Europe and had met two men whom she liked very much. The first one she met in Ireland, where she was staying with her maternal grandmother. It was love at first sight. They had a lovely time together, but, when he proposed marriage, she was a bit surprised and decided to come home to think matters over. As soon as she arrived in Boston, however, she started having second thoughts and soon afterward she wrote to her boyfriend that she was not ready to get married. She dated casually throughout the year while she kept on fighting with her stepfather. The last summer she again went to Europe, but this time she avoided Ireland. She traveled extensively on the continent, met a German student with whom she decided to live for two months, and described having had very satisfactory sexual relations with him. Upon returning to the United States she wrote to him, emphasizing that she had enjoyed their relationship but that she was not interested in making it permanent.

At this point the therapist confronted her as follows:

THERAPIST: Now, there is something peculiar in all this. You tell me that you have only casual relations with men in this country while you fall in love with an Irishman one year and a German the next. The question is, why does the Atlantic Ocean make such a difference as far as your relations with men are concerned?

PATIENT: Oh, come on now, Dr. S! This is silly!

THERAPIST: I'm very serious, even if I put it this way. What strikes me is that there is something special about American men which makes you dislike them, while in contrast in Europe, where you are far away from home, you seem to have perfectly good hetero-sexual relations.

PATIENT: You think that it has to do with my stepfather?

THERAPIST: What do you think?

PATIENT: I think so.

THERAPIST: In what way?

PATIENT: Well, you see, I like my stepfather despite our quarrels. I don't want to "rock the boat" over here, while in Europe it's different.

THERAPIST: So you want to maintain your relationship with your stepfather, who is an American, and thus you avoid getting involved with American men so as not to "rock the boat" and so as not to make him jealous. In Europe, on the other hand, it is different. Somehow you seem to be able to have good relations with men because you are far away from your stepfather.

PATIENT: I have been wondering at times why I stay at home despite these fights with him.

THERAPIST: Because you want the episode at your bed with him when you were twelve to recur.

PATIENT: Oh, no!

THERAPIST: Oh, yes! You know that it is true.

PATIENT (*very thoughtful*): In a way, maybe.

The patient returned the following week saying that things had changed dramatically at home. She did not have a fight with her stepfather. Furthermore, she had met a fellow she seemed to be interested in and had dated him twice.

PATIENT: I've done a lot of thinking about my situation at home and all the things we talked about last week. Do I need any more therapy?

THERAPIST: This is a good question.

PATIENT: Well, I think I understand things very much better.

The therapist, despite the rapid changes which may have been used to escape from therapy, agreed nevertheless that no more therapy was necessary. When seen in follow-up one year later, she had moved away from her parents' home, had no more fights with her stepfather, and was engaged to be married to an *American*.

Who, then, are those individuals who are ripe for a simple psychodynamic confrontation that acts as a catalyst in setting in motion the resolution of their psychological problems? How can we identify them? How many are there in a psychiatric clinic population? Unfortunately, we do not have definite answers to these questions. The experience of Malan and his associates (Malan, Heath, Bacal, & Balfour, 1975) at the Tavistock Clinic in London, where one evaluation interview produced long-lasting beneficial changes, is similar to ours. What is needed is a systematic study which tries to identify those individuals, which describes clearly their psychodynamics, and which specifies how they manage to utilize the psychiatric interview to set in motion the mechanisms which help them rapidly solve psychological problems that have existed over a long period of time.

It is obvious that these individuals have been on the verge of a psychodynamic resolution of their conflicts but have been unable to achieve it by themselves without outside help. It is not necessary that this outside help be professional. A friend, a relative, or even a casual acquaintance may raise a subtle question or make a statement that will set in motion the same problem-solving machinery. But there are also dangers involved in leaving such important matters to chance. Mental health professionals are best equipped, by virtue of their specialized training, to assess and intervene appropriately. We should do all we can to spot these individuals who have a potential to resolve their problems rapidly. One of the difficulties, however, is the incredible speed with which changes can take place in these patients. Psychiatrists who have been trained to believe that psychological reactions take a long time to be modified become suspicious when they see such speedy resolutions and tend to undermine the patient's confidence by implying that they represent a "flight into health" or a "counterphobic reaction," or doubt that the positive results will be maintained. On the contrary, the role of the therapist should be to encourage such patients to do their own problem solving and not to urge them to accept long-term psychotherapy instead.

STAPP does indeed perform such a problem-solving task very quickly. The actual utilization of confrontation and clarification very early, even during the first interview, as we have seen, tends to help the patient come to grips with his own psychological problem. All the additional technical maneuvers which can be used by the therapist will now be discussed in the chapters that follow.

CHAPTER 6

Early Therapeutic Considerations

THE USE OF POSITIVE TRANSFERENCE

It should be emphasized that positive transference feelings usually predominate at the beginning of STAPP. This is primarily due to the extensive work which has been done by the evaluator and the patient and which has given the patient an early taste of what he can expect will take place during the course of therapy. In addition, having a high motivation for change, the patient is eager to settle down and get to work. Because of these factors, therefore, the therapist must discuss with the patient any positive transference feelings which may appear quite early rather than wait for the transference to appear as a resistance and then to interpret it later on. Here is an example:

A 25-year-old social work student started her first STAPP interview as follows:

PATIENT: I was very interested in the way you helped me outline my problem last week. I admired your ability to be so objective. I try to do it with my own clients, but somehow I cannot get the proper distance or the right perspective . . . (*becoming silent*)
THERAPIST: Can you tell me a little more about your feelings for my therapeutic objectivity?

PATIENT: I find it a little embarrassing to talk about you. I was told that one does not bring up . . . (*hesitating*) well, you know, not to use any jargon. . . .

THERAPIST: Go on.

PATIENT: Well, the transference! I was told that the transference must wait.

THERAPIST: Let's talk about your feelings and forget what the books say.

PATIENT: Okay! I did think about you last week after I left. I thought that you had given me much food for thought with your questions. I was grateful for that, because as a result of your interest in my sister and the possible competition between us, I developed a whole new trend of thought. I felt that I wanted you to be on my side.

THERAPIST: Can you tell me more about it?

PATIENT: I have always looked up to Laura (*the patient's older sister*), and I had gone to her many times for advice when I was a teenager. She was very talented. She was the artist, while I was the scientist in our family. She was good at it. I had always thought that our parents appreciated each one of us for our respective talents. When you asked me who was my father's favorite, or, as you put it, "Who was his pet," I felt somewhat surprised because I had not given it much thought. After I left, I felt a little irritated with myself for not having considered or for having dismissed such an eventuality. So I made an effort to remember the times when my father showed some evidence of favoritism and I remembered an episode once when my father had taken all of us out for dinner. My mother suggested that we should have some wine with our meal. I knew that my father drank only beer and that he actually disliked wine. I had always heard him talk about how irritated he felt when the waiters talked to him about wine, about vintages and all that stuff. Laura, I remembered, looked over at the people who were sitting at the table next to us and admired a tall, thin bottle of wine. She said, "Oh, Dad, why don't you order the same bottle these people next to us are drinking from? I can take it home with us and paint it." I said, "Laura, wine is to be tasted, not to be painted." Father took Laura's side. He said, "Of course you should paint that bottle and throw its contents away. For me it's good old Schlitz." Mother intervened at that point and said, "Why don't you have your beer? Kathy and I will drink the wine, and Laura can paint the bottle afterward." I was pleased with mother's support but felt very irritated at Dad. I would have liked him to take my side. Mother's support wasn't enough.

THERAPIST: So, now we see that you wanted me to be on your side in the same way as you wished your father to support you?

PATIENT: That's interesting. I had not thought of it before. Transference, eh!

The patient, being a professional, could easily recognize the transference aspect of her association, yet at first she had missed it. What is striking, however, is her ability so early in the treatment to begin doing her therapeutic work. Her self-inquiry is rewarded by an interesting recollection of an episode that clearly points to her competition with her sister, of which she was unaware.

I have always thought that one must make a distinction between the terms "transference" and "transference neurosis" which, according to Glover (1955), appears during the height of the psychoanalysis of neurotic patients. It is evident, however, that given a certain period of time the transference neurosis eventually develops, even in face-to-face psychotherapy. In such a case, unlike the analyst, who, by virtue of the technique of free associations and frequency of the sessions, has access to all of the patient's fantasies, is able to analyze the transference neurosis, and can terminate the analysis, the therapist, in contrast, is unable to deal with it. He is limited by the weekly face-to-face interaction and the paucity of fantasies. Once a transference neurosis sets in, however, an impasse is reached, and the therapy is prolonged unnecessarily without a clearcut resolution. Thus, time is of the essence in STAPP. The therapeutic work must be done quickly before the transference neurosis makes its appearance. The best way to avoid such an occurrence is to use the patient's transference feelings early. This helps to make the crucial parent–therapist links which create what Alexander and French (1946) call "a corrective emotional experience" and facilitate the resolution of the patient's psychological problem.

Transference is defined as "a psychological interaction between two people having both conscious and unconscious aspects." Transference feelings should be encouraged to develop and must be discussed with the patient as soon as they make their appearance. Here is another example:

A 23-year-old married secretary asked her therapist to give her a prescription for an antihistamine medication which her father, a physician, had once prescribed for her when she had a severe cold:

PATIENT: I seem to have that cold again, and the medicine my father gave me seems to help. Could you give me a prescription for—

THERAPIST (*interrupting*): Can we talk first about your feelings for my giving you—

PATIENT (*interrupting*): Oh, if you don't want to give it to me, I can have my old prescription filled at my pharmacy.

THERAPIST: It is not a question of wanting or not wanting, but rather that I'm interested in your putting me in your father's position. We know that you had very strong and mixed feelings for your father, so I wonder if you have the same feelings for me?

PATIENT: Is that important?

THERAPIST: What do you think?

PATIENT: I don't know.

THERAPIST: Well, let's look at it this way. Your father played a very important part in your childhood. This we discussed already.

PATIENT: That's true.

THERAPIST: Furthermore, there were those boyfriends of yours who had certain characteristics and physical attributes which reminded you of your father, and which you described here last week.

PATIENT: Yes.

THERAPIST: Well, I was just wondering, then, if I also had the same attributes in common with your father.

PATIENT: You are both M.D.s.

THERAPIST: Precisely.

PATIENT: I see . . . there is something in all this.

THERAPIST: Carry on.

PATIENT: My roommate is also in therapy with a psychologist. She and I have talked several times about her treatment, and I remember thinking that I would have preferred to have a therapist who was also a physician. When I was assigned to you, I asked whether you were an M.D. or not. I was pleased when the secretary confirmed that you were. My father is a GP, but he has great respect for psychiatrists.

THERAPIST: So, there is a clear connection in your mind between your father and your feelings for me.

PATIENT: I hadn't thought of it in this connection before, but there is an element of truth in what you say.

At times a patient may try to test the therapist as soon as the treatment begins. Such an opening transference gambit can be difficult to deal with because the therapeutic alliance has not as yet been solidified. Nevertheless, the therapist must discuss these feelings even if he has to take certain chances. Here is an example:

A 26-year-old receptionist had been engaged for a period of three years to a man much older than herself. She had finally decided that she wanted to understand better her relationship with her fiancé in order to make up her mind whether or not to get married.

During the evaluation interview she had emphasized that she had not had sexual relations with him so as not to be "forced" to marry him. She came to her first therapy interview and said:

PATIENT: I thought I should let you know that Bob and I had sexual intercourse last night for the first time. It was quite unsatisfactory.

THERAPIST (*taken aback, but trying to keep calm*): Can you tell me why?

PATIENT: As you know, I did not want to have intercourse because I felt that if I did, I would have to marry Bob.

THERAPIST: Precisely!

PATIENT: Yesterday, however, it seemed to me that now that I was starting therapy I would have the opportunity to discuss everything with my therapist, so I thought, "Why not give it a try?" What do you think? Was it wrong? I ask you as I would have asked my father if he were alive.

THERAPIST: It is not a matter of right and wrong. Furthermore, you are putting me in a position of judging whether what you did is to your advantage. It's not up to me to do this, but rather my role is to help you understand why you do what you do, and for you to decide accordingly.

PATIENT: Yes, that's true.

THERAPIST: Well, not really, because although you decided to marry Bob you ask me what I think about it.

PATIENT: But I haven't decided to marry him.

THERAPIST: Oh, yes you did. You told me that if you had sexual relations with him, and I quote you now, you "will be *forced* to marry Bob."

PATIENT: Yes. I said that, but now I don't feel this way anymore.

THERAPIST: Maybe so, but your action seems to have taken precedence over your understanding. You had difficulty in deciding whether you should marry Bob or not, which you wanted to examine during your therapy. Isn't that correct?

PATIENT: Yes.

THERAPIST: So, you took the bull by the horns and decided that you are forced to marry him. I don't see that there is much for us to do in therapy anymore.

PATIENT: Oh, no! You don't understand. I *do* want therapy. I *do* want to understand. Anyway, it was all very unsatisfactory. I felt that you would be my ally and help me out (*tremulously*), but . . . (*tears*). . . .

THERAPIST: Now you feel sorry for yourself!

PATIENT: Well, yes. You're no help. You don't understand.

THERAPIST: Oh, yes, I do. You don't like what I say, but it's precisely because I want to help you out that I say what I said. Look here, forcing the issue does not solve the problem. Neither does making me the judge, like your father would have been, help you out. What is important is that we both try to understand your conflicts as well as your behavior. Do you want to do that?

PATIENT: Oh, yes. Of course. That's why I'm here.

THERAPIST: Okay, then. First of all, you should stop having sexual intercourse with Bob from now on until we have a clear understanding of what goes on between the two of you. Once we discover that you do want to marry him, and that you are not forcing yourself to do so, then you can resume your sexual relations. As far as I'm concerned, I do not have an opinion as to what you should do one way or the other. My statement should not be interpreted that I take a position against your having sexual relations. It simply means that I am neutral. When *you* decide what you want to do, you can carry on in any way you please.

PATIENT: I do understand now. Okay. I agree.

THERAPIST: One more thing. You said that you were asking me "in the same way as you would have asked your father if he were alive."

PATIENT: Yes.

THERAPIST: Having put me in the position of your father, you present him and me with an accomplished fact. Do you think that your father and I would have approved of your action?

From then on the patient was able to talk at some length about her father and his attitude about sexual relations.

It is obvious that the therapist is put in a difficult position in which he has to deal with the patient's acting-out. Taking a strong position against her continuing to have sexual relations is risky, but he counts on the patient's strong motivation for change to make her decide in favor of understanding and problem solving, even if the therapeutic alliance has not quite been established as yet. Furthermore, he is able to point to a parent–therapist link which he can utilize effectively as the treatment progresses. There is no denying, however, that this is a shaky start and that his statement could have misfired and could have cost him the loss of the patient. Here again one can see the value of a good psychological evaluation and particularly of the importance played by the fifth criterion—the patient's motivation for change—on which the therapist relied completely in this case.

At times because of the patient's resistance to investigate certain Oedipal feelings, the transference may surface during early therapy with such force that it undermines the treatment process. Here is an example of how a therapist successfully handled an early stormy transference situation:

A 22-year-old male freelance photographer was being treated by a female therapist after he had been evaluated in the clinic by two male evaluators. He was late coming to his first interview. Without apologizing, he proceeded to ask his therapist about her professional qualifications. The following exchange took place:

THERAPIST: Why do you want to know about my professional qualifications?

PATIENT: You look very young to me. How many years of training have you had?

THERAPIST: We are not here to discuss my training, but rather your problems. Can you tell me something about them?

PATIENT: Well, okay. (*He went on to describe in some detail his difficulties with his girlfiends which were instrumental in his decision to seek psychotherapy.*) You see, it was my problem with Julie, who was my last girlfriend, which convinced me that I should seek some help. I was very attracted to her, but also I had an urge to pick a fight with her. I also noticed that the more attracted I felt, the greater the need to contradict her, and the worse was the fight which ensued. It was finally Julie who pointed this out to me. She said, "Joe, you're still more attracted to your mother than to any other woman in your life. You don't want to get really close to anyone else. You create these silly fights on purpose. I'm fed up with all this, and I'm going to quit." (*He stopped talking and looked sad.*) You know, the issue about your credentials has not been settled as yet. I have been talking to you about my problem, but you have not answered my question.

THERAPIST: I do not mind answering your question or discussing my training if it's of importance to you, but if it's used to help you avoid talking about your relations with women, or "to pick a fight" with me, then it will not work out in the least.

PATIENT: I see. If I have problems with women, which I admit that I have, then your being a woman may help me sort out these problems.

THERAPIST: It remains to be seen whether you want to be helped or not, or whether you want to repeat the pattern with Julie right here in therapy with me. You know, of course, that there will be no magical cures here. I hope you do.

PATIENT: Yes. I didn't mean that. The two doctors who saw me made it very clear what was expected. I know it's all up to me, but I wonder if a man may be better able to help me.

THERAPIST: First you think that a woman can help you, now it's a man. If there's going to be anyone who can really help you, it is *you*.

PATIENT: Of course.

THERAPIST (*taking a different tack*): Is this the reason why you were late for your first interview?

PATIENT (*taken aback*): Well, I've been thinking about your being a female therapist, but I hadn't planned to be late on purpose. I hadn't actually noticed. Was I late?

THERAPIST: You were exactly eleven minutes late. By the way, I am punctual and I expect you to be on time also.

In the next session the patient was four minutes late. He made no reference to it, but again proceeded to inquire if his therapist had a Ph.D. or an M.D.:

THERAPIST: There we go again! You come late again and you want to talk about my degree.

PATIENT: I was only four minutes late today. I am sorry about that, it just—

THERAPIST (*interrupting*): No apologies, please. If by being only four minutes late instead of eleven you want to indicate that things are improving between us, it's an encouraging sign. You *can* do better than that, however! The question in my mind is whether you are willing to get down to work or not.

PATIENT: Yes, but what do you want me to say?

THERAPIST: It is not what I want you to say, but rather what *you* want to achieve in your therapy.

PATIENT: Last time I was telling you about my difficulties with Julie. (*He again went on to describe his relationship with his last girlfriend in some detail, but when he recounted Julie's confrontation with reference to his mother, he became silent, and soon afterward he again revived the question about having a male therapist*).

THERAPIST: Are you aware of the fact that whenever you touch on the subject of your relationship with your mother you become silent and soon after that you start talking about my credentials or about wanting a male therapist?

PATIENT: No, I wasn't aware of it . . . Hm . . . That's perceptive of you!

THERAPIST: No compliments, please! I'm here to help you solve your problem, at least this is *my* role. I'm not at all sure, however, about your willingness to do the same.

PATIENT: No, no. I do want to understand what happened. I assure you that—

THERAPIST (*interrupting*): Very well then. (*Having felt that her intervention and her challenge had been successful, she went on*): As I mentioned, I do not object to your having questions about my qualifications, or about my being a female, unless you bring them up for the express purpose of avoiding talking about your difficulties with women and your attachment to your mother. I can tell you that I am a qualified therapist on the staff of the psychiatric clinic of this hospital. So, once and for all, I ask you whether you want to work with me or not?

This final and straightforward confrontation and the therapist's willingness to compromise to some degree produced a dramatic effect. The patient was impressed by her skill, by her willingness not to accept any nonsense or to be manipulated, and by her genuine interest in helping him. The treatment proceeded uneventfully from then on.

It should not, however, be forgotten by the therapist that although transference feelings may have been discovered and clarified during the early STAPP sessions, subsequently they may again be suppressed. It is the task of the therapist, therefore, to avoid this by reminding the patient of the transference clarifications which have already taken place. The following example illustrates this point:

MB, a 26-year-old female biologist, started her third STAPP interview as follows:

PATIENT: I have been thinking about our last hour. You seemed to be ahead of me when you said that my interactions with people were very clear-cut. When I left, I thought, "Clear-cut? What does he mean? I am very confused. I don't see anything clear-cut." What I wanted you to do is to tell me, "Go ahead and do thus and so."

THERAPIST: Whom does this statement remind you of?

PATIENT: Oh, clearly this is what mother used to say. She would always give me advice and tell me what to do, but at times her advice irritated me.

THERAPIST: So why did you want me to do something which irritates you?

PATIENT: Well, in this case I would have welcomed the clarification.

THERAPIST: In any case, you wanted me to tell you what to do like your mother used to do.

PATIENT: Yes.

THERAPIST: So you view me like your mother?

PATIENT: Yes.

THERAPIST: But you have told me that you always competed with your mother and with women in general, and that you have always had a "one-up" advantage over them.

PATIENT: Yes, and I also told you about a time when I was seven and I had started to learn how to ski and that I had the fantasy that I would beat my mother in skiing. She was always to be defeated in my thoughts.

THERAPIST: Precisely. So, if you defeat your mother in your thoughts and you view me like your mother, then we must conclude that you wanted also to defeat me.

PATIENT: No.

THERAPIST: Yes. Defeat your therapy.

PATIENT: No, no. Actually, you know, I think of you much more like my father. You are quite well known, as he was. You both have written books. As you know, I read one of your books.

THERAPIST: So, I have features of both your father and your mother.

PATIENT: Yet I could not talk about some of these things that we are discussing here with either of my parents.

THERAPIST: Did you discuss these things with anyone else? With any of your friends, for example?

PATIENT: Oh, I do discuss all these things easily with Bill—you know, my boyfriend.

THERAPIST: So, I have elements of Bill also, in the sense that you can discuss these issues easily with both of us?

PATIENT: Yes.

THERAPIST: So today, summarizing your feelings for me, we can say that there are elements which remind you of your mother, elements which remind you of your father, and elements which remind you of Bill.

PATIENT: In a way this is so.

THERAPIST: So, I am wearing a three-corner hat today!

In the following session the patient discussed some of her feelings about sexuality. She was very anxious and repeatedly expressed the desire that the interview be over so as to escape from her discomfort. Toward the end of the session she said:

PATIENT: By the way, I find it very difficult to discuss the subject of sexuality with you.

THERAPIST: Why with me?

PATIENT: Because you are much older.

THERAPIST: Also because I remind you of your father?

PATIENT: No.

THERAPIST: No?

PATIENT: No. If you remind me of anybody, you may remind me of my grandfather.

THERAPIST: Grandfather?

PATIENT: Well, it is on the tip of my tongue because my grandfather is dead.

THERAPIST: Why do you want to eliminate me in this way? Is it because I am so anxiety-provoking?

PATIENT (laughing): It's that I can't conceive of talking about sexuality with my father or my mother.

THERAPIST: You know that last week we discussed your feelings for me and we saw that there were elements which reminded you of both your father and your mother.

PATIENT: Vaguely I do recall.

THERAPIST: I also had certain aspects which reminded you of your boyfriend, Bill.

PATIENT: I don't remember those.

THERAPIST: What we talked about at the end of the interview last time was the fact that you could discuss certain subjects with Bill in the same way in which you could discuss them with me.

PATIENT: Oh, yes, now I remember.

THERAPIST: Discussion of feelings for your therapist are a very important aspect of this treatment and we should keep that in mind.

PATIENT: OK. I shall.

In this case it is striking to see how anxiety-provoking is the discussion of transference, particularly in the early parts of STAPP.

It is also sometimes remarkable to observe that some STAPP patients have developed fantasies about their therapists and have ready-made expectations about them even before therapy has started and even before they have met them.

Here is an example of a 28-year-old medical student who came for an evaluation interview because of an inability to make up his mind whether or not to accept an offer for an out-of-state job. His procrastination had made him quite anxious.

During the interview the patient mentioned that he was surprised to notice that the therapist did not look at all like his father. He went on as follows:

PATIENT: I have read your articles as a part of my psychiatry course and I had visualized you as being very short and muscular, like my father.

THERAPIST: Are you disappointed that I am not?

PATIENT: No, except when you mentioned that we had to climb two flights up to your office. I thought that you like it this way because it would be good exercise for you to go up and down the stairs. This is what my father does. He keeps in shape and that is why he is so muscular.

THERAPIST: So, how can we understand the fact that in your mind I share certain characteristics with your father, but in reality I look very different from him?

PATIENT: This is interesting because when I first saw you when you called me at the waiting room I thought, "This is not my therapist. It must be a mistake." In a sense I am glad that you are not like my father because I have some conflicts with him, but it is queer that I would feel the way I did about you.

Each patient's defensive maneuvers in reference to the transference feelings for the therapist are diversified to such an extent that, in a cursory discussion of these issues, one can only summarize some of the highlights. Before leaving this subject, however, I should like to discuss briefly a commonly observed defense mechanism involving transference which occurs fairly often with STAPP patients, the early recognition of which by the therapist usually helps to clarify the situation. What I am referring to has to do with a patient who is treated by a therapist of the opposite sex and develops transference feelings that belonged to the parent of the same sex. For example, a female patient may view a male therapist in the early part of treatment like her mother in an effort to avoid displacing onto him her sexualized feelings for her father and experiencing them during the interview. Here is an example:

A 22-year-old female college student had been strongly attached to her father, whome she described as "intellectual and cold" and who, possibly in an effort to avoid his own incestuous feelings for his only child, treated her fairly sadistically, using sarcasm and ridicule and often degrading her in front of other people. He was also very jealous. He disliked her dating partners and once threatened to strike her when she returned late from a date. The patient seemed not to complain about her father's behavior and always acted in a way to please him, even if this gave rise to many difficulties for her. Her relations with her mother were good, and she described her mother as being "warm," "emotional," and "supportive of her." The following exchange took place during the third interview between the patient and the therapist.

PATIENT: I have always tried to please my father. One of the things that made him mad was the time when I showed interest in boys. He always lectured me about all the terrible things that could happen to women, such as rape, pregnancy, and all that, and as I told you last time, once he threatened to hit me.

THERAPIST: What is striking to me is this paradox of trying to please your father when you describe him as being sarcastic and sadistic and—

PATIENT (interrupting): Oh, yes! "Sarcastic" is the word to describe his behavior best.

THERAPIST: If so, why did you try to please him?

PATIENT: As you know, I love my father. I also admire him. He's a genius.

THERAPIST: This may be the case, but why try to please him when he's nasty to you? Are you masochistic?

PATIENT: Well, yes, I am in a way. I remember once when I was quite young I did something wrong, I don't remember what it was, and my father took off his belt and hit my legs and behind. I remember afterward the red marks. It was painful, but I enjoyed the experience. When mother saw the marks, she was very angry with him and told him not to do it again. She was very supportive and soothing to me, but I was very irritated by her behavior, peculiar as this may seem to you.

THERAPIST: Another paradox, eh?

PATIENT: Well, yes . . . . (The patient was silent for a while.)

THERAPIST: You are silent. Why? What are you thinking about?

PATIENT: I felt irritated by your question.

THERAPIST: Can you tell me more about it?

PATIENT: It was . . . in a peculiar way the same kind of irritation that I felt for my mother at that time. This is curious because I know that you're trying to help me and that you're sooth—I mean supportive of—

THERAPIST: You mean soothing like your mother?

PATIENT: In a way that's true. For example, I was thinking, after I left you last time, that psychotherapy was an emotional experience, yet I had pictured it as an intellectual exercise. I had expected an intellectual discussion with you, but, instead, I had one with my girlfriend.

THERAPIST: This is of interest. We know that you view your father as the "intellectual" and your mother as the "emotional supportive" person, yet you have an intellectual discussion with your girlfriend and an emotional one with me, although I am a man. Why do you think that this is happening?

PATIENT: Yes, that's true.

THERAPIST: Why, then, do you have to view me like your mother?

PATIENT: (quiet for a while)

THERAPIST: What thoughts come to mind?

PATIENT: Nothing special . . . (smiling)

THERAPIST: Something must amuse you. You are smiling . . . .

PATIENT: I remembered during the first interview—you know, during that evaluation in front of all those people—what I thought when you were asking me to describe my father. I had the urge to say, but I checked myself . . . that you looked like my father, except for the dark hair.

THERAPIST: Hm! Well, now we have another paradox. A minute ago we observed that you viewed me as your mother, yet during that first interview I reminded you of your father and . . . .

PATIENT((interrupting): I had another thought during that first interview and that's why I checked myself. I thought that, if you reminded me of my father, then I might have the same feelings of trying to please you as I did him.

THERAPIST: So viewing me as your mother is a way of avoiding the feelings that you have for your father.

PATIENT: In a way it's true. I suppose that's why I had an intellectual discussion with my girlfriend.

THERAPIST: Yes, and that's why you wanted me to be soothing and supportive like your mother, and felt irritated at me during this interview as you did with her.

This early transference clarification helped put everything in its proper perspective. As the therapy went on, the patient's sexualized feelings for her father became progressively more apparent and were transferred onto the therapist. Complete resolution of her psychological difficulties was achieved soon afterward. It was clear that her viewing the therapist as her mother in the early part of treatment was her way to avoid dealing with the sexualized feelings for both her father and her therapist, which she explained during the first interview, which threatened her at the time, and which became the motivating force for this defensive transference maneuver.

All this points to one conclusion: "The key to shorter therapy lies in the ability to experience and control the transference," as Alexander (1965, p. 84) put it so aptly.

COUNTERTRANSFERENCE: OCCASIONAL DIFFICULTIES

The feelings of the therapist for the patient are, of course, just as important as the transference feelings for him. Generally speaking, there are few problems involved with countertransference. At times, however, there are some exceptions to this. Here is an example:

A young psychiatric resident had treated a young married woman very successfully and was so pleased with his results that he asked me to supervise his therapy with a second STAPP patient. This was soon arranged for him, and he was assigned to another female patient who had been accepted for our research project, having been found by two independent evaluators to be an excellent candidate.

Following the first interview with his patient, the resident called me to say that he did not think she was a STAPP prospect. I told him not to say anything to the patient before coming for his supervisory session. When I saw him, he told me that he did not like his patient. He went on as follows:

RESIDENT: Dr. Sifneos, this woman is very different from Mrs. M (*the patient whom he had treated successfully*).
SUPERVISOR: Of course, but what difference does it make?
RESIDENT: It does a great deal.
SUPERVISOR: Can you tell me what went on during the first interview?
RESIDENT: Well, yes. I must admit that she has an unresolved Oedi-

pal problem, but she sure is nasty. What problems she has with men! She's a castrating woman!

SUPERVISOR: That is her way of dealing with her Oedipal wishes.

RESIDENT: Maybe so, but boy, what a temper!

SUPERVISOR: Okay, so she has a hot temper!

RESIDENT: She gave me hell. She told me off when I confronted her with her wish to dominate men. What language!

SUPERVISOR: Did you deal with this transference issue?

RESIDENT: Nope.

SUPERVISOR: And why not, since you know it is one of the key technical issues for STAPP and since you dealt with it so well with Mrs. M?

RESIDENT: That's precisely it. She's not like Mrs. M.

SUPERVISOR: Of course not. All STAPP patients cannot be all alike, but look at it this way: Mrs. M also was very angry, but she did not displace it on you. She gave hell to her husband instead.

RESIDENT: Oh, sure she did!

SUPERVISOR: Well, Miss T does, too, but she transfers her anger onto you.

RESIDENT: I can see that, but it's so devastating. It's paralyzing.

SUPERVISOR: Well, that is precisely what you must help her to see so as not to become castrated by her as all her boyfriends have been.

RESIDENT: Okay, I'll see what I can do.

The therapy, stormy at times, proceeded quite well and ended successfully. It was clear, however, that the resident never liked Miss T, but he was pleased to see her work hard and solve her problem. Because of this countertransference difficulty, I was eager to see the patient in a follow-up interview. When I asked her how the therapy had helped her, she went on as follows:

PATIENT: I have solved my problem with men, which is what brought me to the clinic, and this pleases me very much, but I must admit having serious doubts about a successful outcome in the beginning.

EVALUATOR: What do you mean?

PATIENT: Well, at first I did not like my therapist, and I even thought of stopping therapy altogether, but then I said to myself, "Lois, what difference does it make? He is not your boyfriend, he is not your brother, he is not your father. He is trying to help you solve your problem, even if he is a little scared of you. He seems to know what he is doing, so why don't you stick it out and give him a chance? Finish up what you started."

EVALUATOR: And you say that you have succeeded?

PATIENT: Oh, yes, very much so. (*Giving some good examples, she went on to describe how therapy had helped her, how she had resolved her difficulties with men. She was ready to leave when she seemed, on second thought, to have remembered something.*) Dr. Sifneos, one more thing. I told you how I did not like Dr. C very much. Well, this feeling, I think it was reciprocated. I don't think Dr. C liked me very much either!

"Negative transference, negative countertransference, successful outcome!" exclaimed Dr. Fern, a member of our research team, when he heard what I have just described. Indeed, this is, at first glance, a unique experience in psychotherapy, contrary to all the rules. In reality, however, it points to an important observation, namely, that even if the two participants dislike each other, the therapeutic alliance and the common problem-solving goals have an overriding influence on these difficulties and become instrumental in producing a positive result.

It has been said that very little has been written about countertransference by short-term dynamic therapists. This is indeed the case, but it is not at all surprising. Countertransference feelings are of course idiosyncratic and cannot be generalized, but suffice it to say that many therapists like a patient who is making rapid progress in his treatment and who in the final analysis succeeds in overcoming his difficulties. This is precisely what takes place in short-term dynamic therapies in general and STAPP in particular. Therapists who are learning how to treat these patients are surprised at first by their ability to introspect, to problem-solve, and to be inquisitive. They become amazed at the rapidity of their patients' progress, at their insights, at the demonstration beyond any reasonable doubt of the truths about psychodynamics, of the existence of unconscious psychological conflicts, and of the utilization and substitution of maladaptive defense mechanisms with more adaptive ones. Finally, they marvel at the flexibility, honesty, and psychological sophistication of these STAPP patients, particularly if they were to compare them with some of the sicker borderline individuals whom they have treated before. It is difficult not to like some of these patients. That is why few countertransference difficulties are experienced in reference to them.

It is fortunate, however, as already mentioned, that most of the time the countertransference is invariably positive for our STAPP patients.

THE SEX OF THE THERAPIST

The advantages of utilizing evaluators of opposite gender from the patient have already been discussed. The question which must be asked at this point has to do with whether male or female STAPP patients have an easier or a more difficult time with therapists of the same or the opposite sex. From our experience, the sex of the therapist plays no significant role one way or the other as far as the outcome of STAPP is concerned. This conclusion is not surprising, of course, since these patients are individuals who possess considerable strengths of character, who have experience in adjusting easily to frustrating situations, and whose ability to interact well with the evaluator has been carefully scrutinized and has been found to be excellent.

It should not be concluded, however, that the sex of the therapist has no impact on the therapeutic process. On the contrary, the nature of the material that is presented by the patient is clearly connected directly with the sex of the therapist.

For example, male patients who have strong competitive feelings for men that originated from their earlier relations with their fathers tend to avoid bringing up such feelings in their transference for their male therapists. On the contrary, they tend to discuss their heterosexual relations early in their therapy, and the transference material, although generally positive, tends not to appear as early as the therapist may anticipate. When it does appear, it is avoided by the patient as much as possible, because there are some negative aspects to it. It is therefore important for the therapist to keep this in mind, to point to such a resistance as often as possible, and to encourage the patient to talk about some of their competitions.

On the other hand, if these patients are treated by a female therapist, they tend to discuss at length their competition for their fathers and for men in general, while they avoid talking about their sexual feelings for women and their seductive wishes for their therapists.

In either case, however, sooner or later both the competitive feelings for men and seductive feelings for women are dealt with, and considerable insight is gained, even if the timing of their appearance occurs at different times during the treatment.

The same principle applies to female STAPP patients. The strong competitive feelings for their mothers are discussed more easily and earlier with the male therapists, while their sexualized feelings for their therapists tend to be resisted and make their appearance more toward the later part of their treatment. With female therapists, the opposite is true.

It should be emphasized, then, that generally the positive feelings for the therapist tend to predominate.

Despite these difficulties, one may say that the desire of the patients to explore, experiment, and understand is so prevalent, and their motivation and the therapeutic alliance are so strong, that the transference feelings can be described as being on the whole easily dealt with.

It has also been said that it is important that patients should be matched with their therapists and that this is an important nonspecific therapeutic factor in psychotherapy. This may indeed be the case with sicker patients who are receiving long-term supportive psychotherapy, but in my experience over many years of supervising trainees of both sexes in STAPP, I have not found it necessary to transfer patients to other therapists because of a mismatch. From what has been described already, this should not be surprising because STAPP candidates are flexible individuals with a strong motivation to change. They are able to withstand a great deal of anxiety and can adapt themselves to circumstances even if they are not to their liking, such as in the case just described where a negative transference and a negative countertransference predominated.

THE THERAPIST'S "ACTIVITY" IN STAPP

The therapist's "activity" has created considerable controversy since the earliest days of psychoanalysis, particularly after Ferenczi and Rank tried to speed up psychoanalysis by use of active techniques (Ferenczi & Rank, 1925). Ferenczi's new and experimental "active therapy" justified the therapist's activity because it was thought to stimulate the patient's ego sensibility, and, by awakening memories and emotions, it could force from the patient and expose the repressed ideas associated with it. Furthermore, he stressed that interpretation, in itself, is an active interference with the psychic activity (Ferenczi, 1926).

Such departures from classic psychoanalytic technique were at first considered appropriate and justifiable, but the aims to penetrate the deeper layers of the unconscious in a period of a few months and to shorten psychoanalysis were looked upon with suspicion.

It is of interest that Ferenczi actively rewarded and reinforced the patient's associations, using techniques which today are used by behavior therapists.

It is unfortunate, however, that Ferenczi's "active" techniques were pushed to such extreme situations as kissing the patient, to which Freud reacted very strongly.

As far as STAPP is concerned, the activity of the therapist is entirely restricted to making appropriate confrontations and interpretations. The therapist in STAPP is not a "quiet sounding board" or a "passive observer," but neither is the psychoanalyst.

This is possibly understandable because the public has been given the erroneous idea that the psychotherapist is most often a silent sounding board who only on very rare occasions makes noise or utters a few words. This caricature of the psychotherapist may be due to various factors which do not have to be discussed here, but one thing is clear: Behind this silent facade lie his inexperience, passivity, anxiety, conformity, and fear. I do not dispute, of course, that a therapist should listen carefully to what is communicated to him by the patient. This is a *sine qua non* of any form of psychotherapy, but it does not mean that he should limit his activity only to listening. He should be able to make clarifications, ask questions, point out paradoxical attitudes, confront defense mechanisms, and make interpretations explicitly and clearly and, if necessary, repeatedly, until the points have been hammered through and evidence emerges that they have taken hold.

It should be emphasized, however, that even among those who offer short-term psychotherapy there are considerable variations of opinion about the activity of the therapist.

For example, the French and Swiss schools of short-term dynamic psychotherapy generally can be described as being the least active and the most cautious in their interactions with their patients. Malan may also be viewed as being on the less active side, although he uses parent-transference link interpretations extensively. Davanloo, on the other hand, is very active in his broad-focused psychotherapy in an effort to beat down defenses.

In STAPP we also use a very active technique, though not as vigorous as Davanloo's. In many of my workshops I have been criticized as being "aggressive" or of "badgering the patient." I have responded to such criticism by saying that aggression implied hostility, and that this was far from the truth in the case of my countertransference feelings for the patients, but that an active undermining of maladaptive defense mechanisms used by the patient must be systematically pursued in order to help the patient learn to utilize more adaptive patterns of behavior and free himself from his neurotic prison.

The therapist is active in dealing with the transference early, in making patient-transference links, in staying within the Oedipal focus, in avoiding complex pregenital characterological issues, and in helping the patient to problem-solve. Yet all this activity on his part should not be interpreted as implying a lack of sensitivity. On the contrary, if anything, the handling of the transference, for example, signifies that the therapist feels comfortable with the patient and wants to communicate this to him in order to reassure him that, instead of being a threat with his challenges, competitive postures, and strong resistances, he is eager to help the patient deal with the anxieties which he experiences. Above and beyond all other considerations, however, the therapist must convey the fact that he wants the patient to take responsibility for himself, to learn to choose the best way out of a variety of tempting neurotic maladaptive options.

By being active, the therapist also gives something else in return. He is not the passive recipient of the material presented to him by the patient, but, by reformulating it into interpretations, he is able to put it in a different context which facilitates both the understanding and the resolution of the patient's problem once and for all.

This activity, however, is not only limited to anxiety-provoking interpretations. When the therapist witnesses a patient who is struggling to deal with painful material, who is experiencing anxiety, and who is working hard, he should reassure and support the patient as actively as he can.

At this point, I should emphasize that one of the difficulties of STAPP in contrast to other kinds of brief psychotherapy has to do with a tendency on the part of the therapist to ignore, at times, the patient's resistance and proceed to deal with the anxiety-laden content of the material that is avoided by the patient. Putting it in a different way, contrary to the classical psychoanalytic technique of dealing with the defenses first, this approach tends to focus more on the drive or the impulse behind the patient's defense mechanisms. The STAPP therapist, having created a safe environment for the patient to work in by utilizing the therapeutic alliance and positive transference, can afford to be selective and can concentrate on areas in which, in his opinion, most of the patient's conflicts exist—the Oedipal focus. Sensitively paying attention to cues both verbal and nonverbal, he proceeds to expect, and if necessary to demand and to push hard, for painful associations, fantasies, and wishes. In this way, he may succeed in breaking down the resistances. Invariably, when this takes place as a result of his questions, anxiety-provoking confrontations, and clarifications, he is rewarded by the sudden emergence of a fantasy, a dream, or a memory, which pops, so to speak, out of the patient's unconscious and which confirms in a relevant and triumphant way the truth of his interpretations.

MB, the female biologist whose case was described briefly when I discussed transference interpretations in STAPP, was very resistive when we were discussing sexual issues, and she had elevated me to the position of her dead grandfather so as to avoid discussing sexuality with her parents in general and her father in particular. Actually, she had told me in previous interviews that when she was in her adolescence she had had several relationships with men who were much older than herself—about her father's age. At this point the following exchange took place between us:

THERAPIST: Now, as we have seen, you have put me in the position of your grandfather to avoid discussing sexuality with me, yet in the previous interview you had seen me also as a father figure.

PATIENT: Hm.

THERAPIST: But we know already that you had a father who pre-ferred you to your sisters, who was seductive with you, and the effect that this attitude had on you was to make you become in-terested in older men. Isn't that true?

PATIENT: I don't see how that relates to what we have been talking about.

THERAPIST: How come? Didn't you tell me that in your late adoles-cence you had relations with men who were older—about the age of your father?

PATIENT: Yes, we talked about that a long time ago. I don't see why you bring this up now.

THERAPIST: But now we bring it together after all this discussion about sexuality relating to your father. By the way, weren't these rela-tions with these older men sexual?

PATIENT: Yes.

THERAPIST: Well, how is that you say it doesn't relate?

PATIENT: . . . .

THERAPIST: You are silent. What are you thinking about?

PATIENT: In a queer sort of a way I remember an American woman, a friend of mine whom I met when I was in Europe. We were talking about our relation with our parents and I was telling her about my father and describing what we used to do together, and you know what my friend exclaimed? "Oh, you must have had 'a very seductive father.' " I was *aghast*, because I had never thought of it in that way.

THERAPIST: Of course.

PATIENT: Because what I described to her, sitting on my father's lap when I was thirteen, his letting me climb on top of him while driving his car. Yes, all these things were amazing and one could conclude that there was a lot going on between the two of us.

THERAPIST: So you see that it is not all in my head, Dr. Sifneos's head, but also in your American friend's head. She also arrives at the same conclusions. So we can conclude that all these things are true, but that you resist them because they give rise to anxiety. But this example which you gave me despite your resistance was precious evidence that my interpretation was correct.

PATIENT: Yes, this is so.

When they were demonstrated on videotape, these technical

maneuvers shocked many who attended the First International Symposium on Short-Term Dynamic Psychotherapy held in Montreal in 1975. The patient, who was shown in full resistance, did not want to hear what the therapist was trying to confront her with, namely, that she was actively competing with her stepmother in sexual matters. This interpretation was made possible because the patient had repeatedly given information about various events, as well as fantasies and dreams, all of which pointed to her sexual wishes for her father and her feelings of overwhelming superiority in this area over her stepmother, whom she liked nevertheless. The interpretation of the various aspects of her behavior which had been gathered together during the course of her treatment was made early during the eighth interview. The patient tried repeatedly to avoid hearing what was being said by changing the subject. She tried to intellectualize, yet, at the same time, she listened carefully to what was presented to her. Several years later in a follow-up interview, she chose to talk about this particular interview because in her opinion it was the most important one during all her therapy. She said, "I remember how much I disliked what you were saying and how much I tried to stop you because the subject made me so nervous. But I knew all along, in the back of my mind, that what you were talking about was all true and that you were trying to help me, even if I didn't like hearing about it." Such statements point to the importance of the patient's motivation for change, the strength of the therapeutic alliance, and the predominating positive transference.

The therapist, having made a transference interpretation, must be careful to scrutinize its effect during the subsequent therapeutic session. I have seen many patients who furiously resisted my interpretation during the interview only to bring in subsequently a dream, a fantasy, or a memory of an episode which completely confirmed the truth of the interpretation. Here is an example:

A 24-year-old male patient had actively resisted answering the therapist's question about his eight-year-old brother's appendectomy. When asked about his thoughts regarding the appearance of the appendix, he hemmed and hawed, tried to change the subject, talked about the appendectomy in surgical terms, and finally described the appendix as "a hollow organ looking like a stomach or a liver." When I repeated his statement to him, that "the appendix looked like a liver," he looked embarrassed and said, "Well, no, not exactly, maybe it looks more like a worm. It's a useless organ, a few inches long." When asked about its color, he blushed and blurted out that he did not see why all this talk was relevant to his problems.

I actively continued to press him, and because the hour was coming to an end, I told him that I thought that he was resisting discussion of the subject because it made him anxious. I also added that I thought he had a sadistic satisfaction because he viewed the appendectomy as a sort of punishment of his brother inflicted on him by their father. The patient was very relieved that the interview had come to an end and he hurried out of the office as quickly as he could. About an hour later my secretary told me that the patient had called and asked to speak to me. When she asked him what he wanted to talk to me about, he had said, "Never mind, I just remembered something that I thought the doctor ought to hear about, but it's all right, it can wait until next week."

At the start of the next session the patient sheepishly admitted that throughout the previous interview he had the thought that the appendix looked like the penis of a little boy, but somehow he could not bring himself to the point of admitting it, although he realized that it was an important association. He said that, after the hour was over, he felt a bit guilty and thought that I would be disappointed by his performance. It was because of this that he telephoned me. He was relieved, however, when my secretary said that I was not available. As time went by, he felt that he had to admit what his fears were all about. The rest of the hour was spent in exploring in detail his fears of castration and his sadistic feelings for his brother.

It is debatable whether a simple confrontation on the part of the therapist would have produced this turn of events. Rather, it was the therapist's activity, his persistent questioning, and his unwillingness to change the subject that finally gave the patient the clear message of the importance which the therapist placed on this subject. The telephone call, an hour after the interview, was a clear indication to the therapist that he was on the right track.

Here is another example of an interpretation made in face of massive resistance to a 23-year-old male patient during his fourth interview. When the patient was young, he was very much attached to his father, particularly when they went on hunting trips or to baseball games together. After the age of 12 years, however, he started to feel alienated because his father emphasized the importance of studying hard rather than having a good time. On the other hand, his mother was very nice to him during his puberty, and he thought that, because she had been disappointed by the behavior of his older brothers, she had become closer to him.

The patient had felt very upset when his father, a professor of physics at a local university, tried to supervise his homework because he wanted his son to become an engineer. Many fights ensued between the two of them, ending when his mother intervened and took her son's side of the argument. Although he was very bright, he did not do very well in high school, and it was clear that he would not be admitted to the well-known institute of technology his father wanted him to attend. As a result, the father suggested that his son go to a preparatory school. The patient was very angry and refused. As usual he was supported by his mother. Instead, he was accepted at a junior college and majored in liberal arts. His father was very disappointed by this. A compromise was finally reached between the two of them when the patient agreed to take some mathematics and physics courses which might help him if he changed his mind in the future and decided to become an engineer.

The patient did poorly in the junior college and flunked out at the end of his sophomore year, to his father's utter despair. He served in the military for several years and, after his discharge, with the aid of the GI bill, he managed to get a college degree.

He then worked in a large engineering firm and came to the clinic for help because he had some difficulties with his supervisors. He was happily married, had two children, and his relations with his colleagues were very good.

The therapy had concentrated on clarifying his relations with his father and mother. The transference, which was positive, had predominated throughout. Although on many issues the patient was cooperative and worked hard, he always managed to avoid talking about his flunking out of junior college because he claimed he felt very embarrassed by that part of his life. The therapist had thought that this behavior on the part of the patient was an acting-out against his father, but the patient was always resistant when he was confronted with it.

THERAPIST: Now, you never seem to go into detail about flunking out. For example, what were the courses that you failed?

PATIENT: Oh, I don't remember. There were several.

THERAPIST: Now, were these the courses in math and physics that your father wanted you to take?

PATIENT: No. I passed the two math courses. (*The patient proceeded as usual to try to change the subject.*)

THERAPIST: There you go again. We know that you resented your father's checking your homework. We know that you wanted to major in liberal arts rather than become an engineer. We know that you compromised and took some math and physics courses, but you flunked out.

PATIENT: I wanted to be independent. I was bored.

THERAPIST: Yes, but liberal arts was *your* choice, not your father's.

PATIENT (*irritated*): I told you that I passed all the math courses.

THERAPIST: Okay. Now, if you wanted to be independent, why did you flunk out in the courses that you chose? Furthermore, doesn't it strike you as somewhat peculiar that you are now working in a large engineering firm, which is what your father always wanted you to do?

PATIENT: Yes, Dad's pleased that I have given up the idea of doing something in the field of liberal arts.

THERAPIST: So how can we explain all this?

PATIENT: Just coincidence.

THERAPIST: Come now, you know better than that.

PATIENT: Fine, so what do you want me to say?

THERAPIST: I don't want you to say anything. I am, I mean *we* are interested in trying to figure all this out, as we have already done so many times during this treatment.

PATIENT: Yes, I know, but there's nothing more in all this.

THERAPIST: Now, you are resisting talking about this subject.

PATIENT: It's because I don't think there's more to be said about it.

THERAPIST: Yes, there is, and you know it. Now, you say you passed the math courses. Which courses did you flunk?

PATIENT: I don't remember. There were one or two courses I got an F in. I took the exam again, and again I got an F. They sent me a final warning and again I failed. So they asked me to leave.

THERAPIST: What was that course?

PATIENT: I draw a blank.

THERAPIST: You do because you want to run away from it.

PATIENT: Maybe.

THERAPIST: You keep on emphasizing that you passed all the math courses. What about the physics courses?

PATIENT: Oh, maybe that was the course I flunked. Come to think of it, I remember all of a sudden that it was in physics.

THERAPIST: Why?

PATIENT: Well, I just couldn't concentrate. I couldn't study; that textbook was so dull, so boring.

THERAPIST: Textbook?

PATIENT: Yes . . . (blushing)

THERAPIST: Can we hear about it?

PATIENT: That's about it.

THERAPIST: Don't run away.

PATIENT (sheepishly): Well, it was a physics textbook that my father had written.

THERAPIST: I see!

PATIENT (his voice becoming tremulous): Well, was that what you wanted to hear?

THERAPIST: Now, as I said before, it's important that you look at all this and understand what went on. I am not here to help you confess your sins, neither am I here to enjoy your discomfort. I am here to help you understand yourself so as to overcome your difficulties—

PATIENT (interrupting): I know that, doctor.

THERAPIST: Okay, now we can see all these events in an entirely different way.

The therapist proceeded to recapitulate, and the interview ended in a positive way. In a follow-up interview the patient remembered this session as being the most important one of his course of therapy.

An example of an early STAPP interview will be presented in the next chapter to demonstrate the early phase of this therapy.

CHAPTER 7

An Example of an Early STAPP Interview

Before describing the height of the treatment process, I would like to give in some detail a typical STAPP interview during its early phase.

The patient is a 28-year-old male teacher complaining of difficulties in his relationship with his wife. He described his problem as follows: "My wife directs her anger at me and at our kids all the time. I am fed up with it. She used to be sullen and withdrawn, but lately, ever since she started seeing a psychiatrist, she has changed her behavior. She has become aggressive, claiming that I do not support her, that I do not satisfy her needs, and that I am not interested in her sexually. This latter point is partly true, but it's more as a result of her attacks on me. Recently I have felt quite tired and on several occasions I had a premature ejaculation, which didn't help matters and which infuriated my wife."

The patient was the oldest of three children. He had two younger sisters. He was clearly the favorite of his mother, who, as a result of her constant fights with her highly successful businessman husband, used to complain to her son about her husband and tried to make him her ally. As a result, he felt always in the middle of a battle, and he resented his mother's attempts to use him in order to manipulate her husband. Yet, at the same time, he experienced a "strange satisfaction" at being in that position. He liked and admired his father, particularly when they had intellectual discussions together. The patient did brilliantly at college and had an excellent teaching job at a well-known university.

He fulfilled all the criteria for selection for STAPP, and the Oedipal focus was clearly in evidence.

His therapy proceeded quickly and uneventfully during the first three interviews. The positive transference feelings were expressed openly to the therapist, particularly when he compared the treatment with the "enjoyable intellectual discussions he had with his father." Furthermore, he saw a clear parallel between his mother's angry outbursts when he refused at times to manipulate his father and his wife's aggressive behavior when he refused to satisfy her needs.

The following exchange took place during the fourth interview:

PATIENT: I was dazed after I left you last week, particularly as a result of clearly seeing that my mother and my wife have certain characteristics in common which I had never realized before. Furthermore, I thought of another aspect of my wife's behavior which reminded me of my mother's. You see, Bonnie (*his wife*) really has the same puritanical attitude about sex as my mother. I remember that when I was fifteen my mother told me that she thought my father related to me the same way as he did with his younger brother, with whom he also had intellectual conversations. She also said, "I think it's silly for a grown-up man to deal with his son as if he were his brother . . ." (*The patient smiled at this point.*)

THERAPIST: I notice that you smile. Why?

PATIENT: I remember something else that mother said.

THERAPIST: What was that?

PATIENT: On another occasion my mother called me by my father's name. She seemed embarrassed and added that she "didn't want to make me into a husband."

THERAPIST: So, if your mother viewed you as "a husband," how did your father feel about it?

The therapist has chosen the option of inquiring about the feelings for the father, which he felt were more promising to pursue since the material about the mother was easily brought into the open by the patient.

PATIENT: Oh, well, my father was jealous of me. I know this because at such times his ability to discuss intellectual issues with me would become impaired. I would notice flaws in his logic, which was very unusual because he was very smart. I knew then that he was emotionally upset.

THERAPIST: And how did you feel about that?

PATIENT: Both proud, but also uneasy.

THERAPIST: So competition with your father makes you uneasy.

PATIENT: Yes, but I don't give up. My father has a factory, and during the summers I used to work for him. But I remember we used to get into fights so often that when I became eighteen I told him that I didn't want to work for him anymore and that I was going to get another summer job.

THERAPIST: So you became independent!

PATIENT: Yes. Actually I got paid much less money, but I was my own boss.

THERAPIST: And you felt good standing on your own two feet?

PATIENT: You bet. I was proud, very proud! (*He was quiet for a while and then, changing the subject, he went on:*) A sexual thing jumped into my mind.

THERAPIST: Go on.

PATIENT: On two occasions in my life I've seen my mother accidentally without her clothes on. It troubled me and I was curious. I remember clearly her breasts and her pubic hair . . . (*He became silent at that point.*)

THERAPIST: And how did you feel about it?

PATIENT: I felt troubled.

THERAPIST: Troubled?

PATIENT: Yes, because my mother had once said that children tend to love one parent more than the other and that she hoped I loved her more than Dad.

THERAPIST: Did you?

PATIENT: Well, sort of, but I lied and I said that I loved them both equally.

THERAPIST: Why did you lie?

PATIENT: Because I felt uneasy. If I said that I liked her more, I was worried about what my father would do.

THERAPIST: You mean if he found out that you were curious about seeing her naked?

PATIENT: Hm. I hadn't thought of it this way. I was thinking more about this "love choice," but come to think of it, you may have something there.

The therapist by his insistence on getting information about the patient's competition with his father becomes aware belatedly that he may be missing some interesting associations in reference to the mother. The patient's willingness to agree with him too readily makes him suspicious, so he proceeds as follows:

THERAPIST: Yet you used the word "troubled" in referring to seeing your mother naked. What were you "troubled" about?

PATIENT: Yes, "troubled" is the right word, because I feel troubled when Bonnie makes sexual advances on me.

THERAPIST: Can you tell me more about this "troubled" feeling?

PATIENT: Well, the other day Bonnie wanted to have intercourse. She started to take her clothes off. At first I felt excited, but then I became apprehensive. She noticed my expression and started to make some derogatory remarks. I felt angry at her and I had a premature ejaculation. After that she was furious.

THERAPIST: So you felt troubled?

PATIENT: Well, yes.

THERAPIST: What comes to mind?

PATIENT: My mother's tirades at my father. She used to emasculate him so. (He was silent for a while.)

THERAPIST: You are silent. What are you thinking about?

PATIENT: I have a peculiar feeling of wanting to be a little boy.

THERAPIST: What about this feeling? Can you tell me more about it?

PATIENT: It has to do with my father. He was so successful in business, as I have already told you.

Since the patient now associates to his father, a subject which he avoided before, the therapist thinks that he is trying to avoid talking about his sexual feelings for his mother, so he proceeds as follows:

THERAPIST (*interrupting*): Does it really have to do with your father, or is it possibly more a way to deal with your troubled feeling in reference to your mother?

PATIENT: Well, my mother always admired my physique. That's what really troubled me.

THERAPIST: Go on.

PATIENT: She used to inquire so much about my dates. She didn't want me to date. You know, I had plenty of opportunities to have sexual intercourse, but I didn't before I was married. I wanted to be a master at it and I was afraid that I would be inadequate.

THERAPIST: But if your mother admired your physique, why were you afraid that you'd be inadequate in sex, unless of course—

PATIENT (*interrupting*): Intercourse would be a threat to her.

THERAPIST: To her or to you?

PATIENT: (*silence*)

THERAPIST: Is this why you feel like being a little boy? Is this a way to avoid having sexual feelings, "troubled" feelings for your mother?

PATIENT (*looking quite anxious*): My mother used to lecture me about sex. "Sex saps your energy," she used to say. "Don't overdo it. Don't begin to be interested in girls too early."

THERAPIST: Is this then why you conserved your energy and have a premature ejaculation with your wife when she has angry outbursts like your mother?

PATIENT: Hm! I never thought of it before. It sure makes sense!

THERAPIST: Do you want to be a little boy to avoid all these sexual problems, both with your wife and with your mother?

The interview went on for a while longer, the patient reminiscing about various aspects of his relations with his girlfriends, his desire for them, and his fear that if his mother found out about it she would be angry.

It is clear that during this interview the patient is resisting talking about his sexual desire for his mother. Rather, he prefers to be evasive. The fear of his father's reaction is also avoided, and the need to be a "little boy" offers him a way out of talking about his desires for his mother. It is clear, however, that he works hard during the interview and can see clearly the similarities between his mother and his wife, as well as the meaning of his symptom—

which has played an important role in his seeking psychotherapy—i.e., his premature ejaculation following his wife's angry outbursts. All in all, this interview points out how fast STAPP can proceed with a suitable patient. It should be remembered that this is only the fourth interview.

It should be pointed out that the rapidity with which STAPP patients proceed, and their eagerness to bring in a great deal of material during the early part of therapy, has a tendency to frighten trainees who have been taught by long-term psychotherapy advocates that it takes a great deal of time for such material to surface, and therefore they tend to become suspicious of these early and significant associations of their STAPP patients.

It should of course be kept in mind that some patients may produce so much material in order to flood their therapists with it, as a form of resistance. This type of reaction is, however, very different from the kinds of issues which I have just described. In any case, if too many associations are brought up by the patient as a form of resistance, they very rarely are associated with the focus which has been specified and agreed upon by both patient and therapist. If this is the case, the best thing for the therapist to do is to interrupt the patient, remind him that he has deviated from the focus, and urge him to divert his attention and his associations to it.

At this point all the preliminary preparatory work has been accomplished. Now the treatment is about to reach its height.

CHAPTER 8

The Height of STAPP

The therapist should keep clearly in mind the following technical aspects of STAPP which have similarities to, and differences from, other kinds of brief therapy when he selects an appropriate candidate and, after the opening phase, when he is rapidly reaching the height of this treatment.

THE THERAPEUTIC FOCUS AND THE OEDIPUS COMPLEX

Much has been said already about the therapeutic focus during the discussion of the patient's evaluation, and this should be recalled because it plays a key role at this stage of the therapy.

As a result of our outcome studies, we were able to ascertain that the best results were obtained with patients whose problems were clearly Oedipal in nature. Therefore, we decided to concentrate our investigation on these individuals so as to understand better the nature of their difficulties and thus be able to develop the short-term therapy best suited to their idiosyncratic needs.

Over the last few decades, Oedipal conflicts seem to have been downgraded in importance as far as the psychiatric literature is concerned, and a great deal of attention seems to have been placed on understanding early oral and other pregenital difficulties, particularly as seen in seriously disturbed individuals. This is possibly a

however, with well-circumscribed problems seem to have been ne-
glected. Why should that be? Why should so little attention be
placed on the Oedipus complex, this universal and formidable
problem which has plagued man for so long, and which has had
such a profound and dramatic impact on him at least since the days
of Sophocles? I think the answer to this question can be found in
the unresolved or partially resolved psychological conflicts of the
therapists themselves. As I mentioned earlier, not only is the uni-
versality of the Oedipal complex well known, but also the many difficulties encountered in its resolution. It is easier for the therapist,
therefore, to concentrate on earlier and more ancient kinds of difficulties such as the oral ones, which are far removed from his own
consciousness, than to deal with his own Oedipal anxieties, which
STAPP patients present very vividly to him, and which are much
closer to the therapist's immediate awareness.

There are, of course, considerable individual variations in the
handling of Oedipal problems which become the therapeutic focus
of STAPP. However, in order to generalize, one could exaggerate
and say that in a female patient an actual rejection by the father at
the time of her heightened Oedipal wishes for him has a more det-
rimental effect on her psychopathology than the decision on the
part of the patient to give up her longings for her father voluntarily
and search for a substitute, so as to avoid the guilt feelings resulting
from her competition with her mother.

The actual rejection of a daughter by her father, for whatever
reasons, gives rise to a narcissistic wound which, although not
devastating, nevertheless adversely affects the daughter's self-image
as well as her self-esteem. The resulting anger from the realistic or
fictitious parental rejection is somewhat more difficult to deal with
during therapy than the sadness which results from the voluntary
abandonment of the father in order to arrive at a peaceful compromise with the patient's mother.

Similar conflicts do take place with males, but the nature of the
competition with their fathers is more open and the anger appears
to be closer to the surface, more accessible, and easier to handle
during the treatment. In male cases, therefore, one encounters
fewer guilt feelings predominating than is the case with females
competing with their mothers. Guilt feelings may not be as pre-
dominant, but fears about castration play an important part in the

psychodynamics of male patients. Malan questions whether one should interpret such castration fears during brief psychotherapy. From our experience with STAPP males, the answer is categorically affirmative. The castration fears are interpreted because they are used defensively by the patient to present himself as a victim so as to deceive his father in order to avoid his potential competition with him. Homosexual fears also fall in the same category. In my book on short-term psychotherapy (Sifneos, 1972), I described a case of anxiety and homosexuality in which such feelings were clearly used defensively by the patient to pacify his father and to pretend, by giving the false impression of being a homosexual, that he had no heterosexual wishes for his mother.

In addition, the aggressive wishes of the patient to castrate others should also be interpreted, and this can best be done within the context of transference. This will become clearer when I discuss the avoidance of pregenital characterological issues. It should not be forgotten, however, that what is important are the subtle individual ways in which each patient approaches his or her Oedipal wishes. These idiosyncratic variations are responsible for making STAPP so diversified and so exciting.

Of course, what plays a key role and predetermines the nature of the Oedipal struggle has to do with the pregenital character development of the patient. STAPP candidates usually have experienced no serious problems before they were confronted with the difficult Oedipal choice. This is why considerable time must be spent during the evaluation to ascertain that this indeed was the case. Thus, the best evidence of a healthy early development is the demonstration of the existence of a "meaningful" relationship during early childhood.

If STAPP patients encountered no major obstacles while they were growing up, then one must find out the reasons why, during their Oedipal period, they faced certain difficulties which interfered with the resolution of their psychological problem. From our experience, it appears that indeed some major specific external event took place which complicated the choice of a heterosexual partner. For example, a female patient may have had an overly seductive father while the mother may have been equally exhibitionistic with her son. On the other hand, the parent with whom the patient was competing might have been absent for a long time, leaving the field result of the general tendency of the majority of therapists to treat such patients over long periods of time. The healthier patients, open to them, so to speak. Such realistic events tend to tempt the patient excessively and play a role in delaying his choice for a parental substitute, while he maintains the attachment to the heterosexual parent. The actual preference for another sibling by a parent also gives rise to jealous feelings, complicating the successful Oedipal resolution.

All these considerations must be kept in mind by the therapist who focuses on these triangular relations during STAPP, and who should be prepared to become the recipient of the transference feelings which belonged to the parent of the same sex as the therapist.

One of the most interesting aspects of handling the Oedipal therapeutic focus has to do with what is referred to as "splitting."

This type of splitting has no connections of course wih the "splitting" utilized by borderline patients and which is very familiar to therapists who treat them. The Oedipal splitting observed in STAPP involves the patient's displacement of his positive desires onto two or more individuals, while the negative feelings are projected onto different surrogates. For example, a young female patient described at length being her father's favorite up to the age of six years. She remembered with great relish his teaching her how to dance. An ecstatic smile appeared on her face as she recounted her father's admiration of her when she wore her ballet dress and danced Tchaikovski's *Swan Lake* for him. As she grew older, however, her relationship with her father cooled down considerably. Although she could not explain exactly why this happened, she did think that it might be associated with the birth of her younger sister when she was seven years old. She was very precise, on the other hand, about two memories. The first one had to do with the constant fighting which took place between herself and her older brother, who on several occasions did some baby-sitting for their parents. This brother was eight years her senior. He was cruel and on many occasions used his physical strength to abuse here. She remembered with much anger being pinned down on the floor by him. She flushed when she described how he had put his knees on her arms, while he sat on top of her and slapped her face until she had a nosebleed. After she managed to extricate herself from his grasp, she ran to her uncle's house across the street while she was still bleeding. Her uncle was very supportive. The second memory was associated with the development of a very close relationship to this uncle, who on many occasions had fondled her. In this way she was able to split the Oedipal feelings which she had experienced for her father into two directions: the positive ones were displaced onto her uncle and the negative ones onto her brother.

This shifting, splitting, and displacing of feelings onto various members of the family occurs most often in patients who come from large families where it is easy for the child to get what he wants by going around from one family member to another. At times, however, even a single child can find gratification of his wishes by going around to neighbors and friends of the parents so as to split his Oedipal feelings, thus making them easier to deal with.

THE USE OF ANXIETY-PROVOKING QUESTIONS, CONFRONTATIONS, AND CLARIFICATIONS

The best technical tools available to the therapist to enable him to remain on the therapeutic focus are the use of questions and confrontations timed appropriately and aimed at creating enough anxiety to maintain the patient's motivation for problem solving on a high level (Adler & Myerson, 1973). Here is an example:

A 24-year-old male patient had talked during the first three interviews of his therapy about his closeness to his mother. He was the youngest of several children and was clearly his mother's favorite child. He remembered how she referred to him as her "last baby." He recalled his mother's saying to him when he was five years old that she was sad because he had grown up so fast that he could not fit on her lap anymore. One of his fondest memories had to do with the days when his mother did the washing. The transference predominating during these first few interviews was of a positive nature and had been clarified on several occasions. The following exchange took place during the fourth interview:

THERAPIST: What was so fascinating about "washing day"? You mentioned this interest of yours before. We also know that it has something to do with your feelings for your mother.
PATIENT: Oh, yes, indeed! It was wonderful to be with Mom. I

always remember how she asked me to bring down all the dirty clothes. Then I would watch her sorting them out into these neat piles. Of course, I was most fascinated by all those feminine things that belonged to her and to my older sister . . . all the lingerie, nightgowns, stockings, panties . . . (*smiling*)

THERAPIST: Go on.

PATIENT: It was all so exciting, so much fun. It was such a "warm" feeling I had for my mother. (*He went on describing various details about "washing day," and then associated, smiling again, to his "sexual" arousal about certain undergarments of his wife's. Soon afterward, however, he returned to the subject of his mother's "washing day" and again described the "warm" feeing he had for her.*)

THERAPIST (*interrupting him*): You mean "sexual" feeling.

PATIENT (*taken aback*): No, I said "warm" feeling.

THERAPIST: Oh, yes, I heard you very well. You said "warm." It was I who used the word "sexual" because sexual was the right term, and you were using "warm" to dilute that feeling for your mother.

PATIENT (*somewhat irritated*): I can use any word I wish.

THERAPIST: Of course, but if certain words tend to obscure the real meaning or the real feeling, then it's important that I bring it to your attention. You see, it was you who talked about your "sexual arousal" by certain undergarments that belonged to your wife. The word "sexual" was appropriate to your feelings for your wife, yet for the same undergarments being washed by your mother you chose to emphasize the "warm feeling." Now, I don't see why the same female undergarments should produce different kinds of feelings in you unless you felt that it was inappropriate to talk about sexual feelings for your mother. Is it true?

PATIENT: Well, sort of.

THERAPIST: No "sort of." Yes or no?

PATIENT (*blushing*): Well, yes.

THERAPIST: Of course! But you see, it was quite evident that it was so, because when you were describing all your mother's undergarments, you said you were fascinated by them, and when you mentioned the specific items, you started to smile. Later on, while you were describing your "sexual arousal" at your wife's undergarments the same smile again appeared on your face. So I knew that "sexual" was what you were thinking about in reference to your mother instead of "warm," but the word "sexual" was loaded. It was much more anxiety-provoking so you decided to substitute another, more innocuous word. Your smile gave it away!

The proper timing of such confrontations is of importance, but the therapist must also be careful to substantiate such anxiety-provoking technical interventions with all the evidence that he has amassed while listening to the patient's associations and recollections. An element of surprise always helps the proper timing of the therapist's confrontations and clarifications, because it has a greater impact on the patient. The evidence that the therapist's intervention has had an effect should be gauged not only by the words that are being spoken, but also by observation of sudden shifts in the patient's associations, slips of the tongue, uncomfortable silences, blushing, inappropriate facial expressions, or finally, postural changes.

Generally speaking, the questions most likely to produce anxiety are invariably associated with material from the Oedipal focus, or from transference feelings. Therefore, these are used repeatedly by the therapist to make the all-important therapist–parent connections or links (to be discussed in more detail later), because they have been shown to play a vital role in the success of all brief psychotherapies.

I have always emphasized that, in order to be effective, confrontations or clarifications must be painful to a certain degree so as to help facilitate the process of self-understanding and keep the patient's motivation at a high level. By virtue of his position as an impartial outside observer who is not involved with the patient's psychological conflicts, the therapist is well suited to confront the patient with paradoxical situations, illogical conclusions, ineffectual responses, irrational wishes, and maladaptive behavior patterns, all of which may not be appreciated immediately by the patient but are nevertheless true.

All this may be interpreted as being unusually harsh. There is a reality to this conclusion, but since the therapist has the patient's best interest in mind, he must risk creating a certain degree of discomfort to achieve his therapeutic task. Furthermore, I consider it complimentary to think that the patient has the strength to withstand a certain discomfort in order to achieve a superior level of psychological adjustment.

Is there a danger that the therapist may use confrontation to satisfy his own sadistic needs? I shall discuss this later (in the chapter on supervision), but it can be stated at this point that rarely, if ever, is this the case. On the contrary, I have been impressed more by the opposite attitude on the part of the therapist, namely, a tendency to be unusually gentle because he does not have full confidence in the strengths of the patient, or in his own ability to assess it correctly. Such an attitude, emanating possibly from the therapist's omnipotent self-importance, tends to make him think that he is indispensible to the patient and again helps prolong the treatment unnecessarily.

THE PAST-TRANSFERENCE LINKS

The advantage of making these links is obvious because it brings into the therapeutic relationship the old Oedipal problems and all the feelings associated with them. It gives the patient and the therapist the opportunity to examine all these factors and feelings, so to speak, "alive" during the interview.

Thus the opportunity to create an atmosphere in which an improved psychological interaction, or "a corrective emotional experience," as Alexander and French (1946) have called it, can take place is made available to both members of the therapeutic relationship. The displacements onto the therapist of the feelings, attitudes, and behavior patterns which the patient experienced for the parent of the same sex can be examined, clarified, and analyzed. The possibilities for the development of new learning, of novel patterns of behavior, are made available to the patient. For in the final analysis the resolution of the basic Oedipal problem depends on the new learning and cognitive understanding, and successful utilization of the insights which have been achieved, as well as the experiencing of the feelings which have been aroused during the therapy as a result of the interpretations associated with these therapist–parent connections. Here is an example:

A 24-year-old male graduate student had spent a great deal of time during the first few interviews talking about his attachment to his mother, while he had barely mentioned the existence of his traveling salesman father. At the height of his therapy, transference feelings for the therapist had not yet appeared. It was after the therapist was absent for 14 days that the patient talked in detail about the events of the previous weeks. Finally the following exchange took place:

PATIENT: I missed our sessions during the past two weeks.

THERAPIST: Can we talk about it then?

PATIENT: There is not very much to say, except that I like my sessions and I look forward to coming here and exploring my feelings. Last week when the time came for my hour and I remembered that it was canceled, I felt somewhat sad. I was wondering what you were doing.

THERAPIST: Yes?

PATIENT: I didn't think that you were on vacation. Actually, I knew that you were not on vacation, because I overheard a doctor who was talking to someone else in the corridor mention that you were going to Europe for a professional lecture tour.

THERAPIST: So you know.

PATIENT: Yes, I do, but of course I don't know where you were going or what exactly you were doing.

THERAPIST: Does all this remind you of anything?

PATIENT: In a strange sort of a way, it reminds me of my father. As you know, he was a traveling salesman. I remember once that my brother John had mentioned that Dad was going to Alaska to sell some machinery. John was quite excited about it, because he thought that Alaska was a fascinating place. He said that Dad would have a lot of stories to tell us about his adventures over there after he returned, all about polar bears, other wild animals, and all that. John also reminded me that he was going to be the "man of the house" while my father was away, because he was the oldest.

THERAPIST: How old were you?

PATIENT: I was eight and John was twelve.

THERAPIST: How did *you* feel about your father's trip?

PATIENT: I was used to his trips, but I remember that I thought Alaska was too far away and two months was a very long time for Dad to be away. I felt kind of sad.

THERAPIST: So, there is a connection between your father's and my trip.

PATIENT (*somewhat surprised*): How come?

THERAPIST: You said that you felt sad last week at the time of our session, and you had the same feeling about your father's trip. (*The therapist takes an opportunity to make a therapist–parent link.*)

PATIENT: Yes, I see what you mean. There was something interesting that happened later on. My father had to postpone his trip because John got sick the night before he was going to leave, and they had to take him to the hospital. I was terrified of hospitals because my father had taken me there to have several stitches in my leg when I fell off my bike. I also remember that my sister Sally had her tonsils out in that same hospital. (*At that point it was the end of the hour.*)

THERAPIST: I'm intrigued because you spent so much time at the beginning of the hour talking about all the details of the last two weeks, and only in the last few minutes did you start talking about some important feelings in reference to me which are similar to those that you had for your father. Maybe we can continue to talk about all this next time.

The patient came the following week, saying that he had done a great deal of thinking during the intervening time:

PATIENT: I have thought about what you said at the end of last week's session, about feeling sad about my father's Alaska trip and about your European lecture tour. I had also a dream the following night. I had come to your house and you greeted me with a smile. We had our interview in your dining room. Your daughter came in and you said, "Hi, Cathy, take Mr. W to the garden." She looked at me and invited me to go along with her. I got up and left, although the hour wasn't over, but then I felt apprehensive because I thought that you would be mad at me, so I came back. The door was locked and you were gone, so I took your car. I drove very fast, looking all over for you, but I couldn't find you, and then I had a crash. I was injured and bleeding. You soon appeared and took me to the hospital with your ambulance. I remember pleading with you not to take me there, but you said we had to go because otherwise I might die. At that point I woke up I was in a cold sweat!

THERAPIST: An interesting dream! Let's hear your associations to it.

PATIENT: There were the obvious similarities with what we were talking about last week.

THERAPIST: Indeed! Now what was the most important part?

PATIENT: The hospital part, John and Sally having been there. My stitches and my pleading with you not to take me there.

THERAPIST: Precisely, but I do take you there in the dream.

PATIENT: Yes, you do, and I'm terrified.

THERAPIST: But you came back looking for me. Why?

PATIENT: I was scared.

THERAPIST: *Why?*

PATIENT: Because I felt guilty about leaving you and going away with Cathy.

THERAPIST: Now what about Cathy?

PATIENT: The queer thing about it is that there is no reason why I should have felt guilty, because you seemed to have told her to take me out in the garden.

THERAPIST: Hmm!

PATIENT: There was something peculiar . . .

THERAPIST: Yes, you said the "queer thing was" . . . What was so queer in all this?

PATIENT: Well, she seemed to be much older. Actually, she couldn't have been your daughter because she looked more like a forty-year-old woman.

THERAPIST: I see! Now what about all this?

PATIENT: . . . She could have been your wife.

THERAPIST: So, you abandon me and go away with my wife, eh?

PATIENT: *You* send me away.

THERAPIST: That's what happens in the dream, but why do you feel apprehensive then and have to come back looking for me?

PATIENT: To be honest with you, the feeling was more one of guilt than apprehension.

THERAPIST: Guilty feelings imply that some crime has been committed. We know that you view your going to the garden with Cathy as an act that was going to make me mad.

PATIENT: Yes.

THERAPIST: Let's go back to Cathy. You said that she looked like a forty-year-old woman. Did she remind you of someone else?

PATIENT: The queer thing is—

THERAPIST: There are a lot of "queer" things going on today.

PATIENT: Well, yes, because she looked, come to think of it, like
—(hesitating)

THERAPIST: Go on.

PATIENT: Like my mom.

THERAPIST: So you went with your mother and abandoned your father!

PATIENT: No, I abandoned you in the dream.

THERAPIST: Come now! You forgot already what you said at the beginning of the hour, and also what we saw so clearly last week—that you view me like your father.

PATIENT: Yes, I see.

THERAPIST: Furthermore, all the evidence in the dream points to that direction, because I take you to the hospital as your father did.

PATIENT: It's amazing how the human mind works!

THERAPIST: It is true, but it's strong in the area of the marvels of *your* mind. Can we recapitulate what we know?

PATIENT: Yes, I guess so.

THERAPIST: No guesses. Do you or don't you want to know. After all, it was *your* dream. I was not there. You introduced me.

PATIENT: Yes.

THERAPIST: So, as we know, you wanted to take Cathy, who was like your mother, away from me, who reminds you of your father. This wish, of course, terrified you because you were afraid that I, like your father, would be angry with you. So you come back, but quickly you manage to become the victim and to be taken to the hospital, which you view as a punishment.

With these clarifications the therapist was able to utilize the therapist–parent connection which he had made during the previous session to bring together the patient's wishes for his mother, the therapist's wife-daughter, and his fears of retaliation in the form of castration by the therapist-father. The psychodynamics of the patient's Oedipal focus were clearly understood by the end of that hour, which was only the fifth therapeutic session. The dream, emanating straight out of the patient's unconscious, provided invaluable evidence, which was effectively utilized to pinpoint the therapeutic focus and initiate the beginning of new learning which contributed to the eventual resolution of the patient's problem.

Of all the technical aspects of short-term dynamic psychotherapy, the ability of the therapist to make links with feelings which the patient had for his parents or parental surrogates, with feelings which are transferred onto him during the therapy, is probably the most important of all the technical tools being utilized. Malan has paid special attention to these links and has correlated them with successful outcome based on sophisticated dynamic criteria (Malan, 1976c).

Here is an example of how a past-transference link can be utilized in STAPP.

MB, the young female biologist whose interactions with the therapist have been discussed in reference to her transference feelings for him (p. 100), when the subject of her sexuality came up, emphasized that she wanted to end the sessions early because of her intense anxiety. Up to that point during the therapy the patient had been dressing like a little girl, in an almost inappropriate fashion. She came to the following session dressed in a very grown-up way, almost as if she were going to go out for dinner. She started the session as follows:

PATIENT: After last week's hour, when I left I was so anxious that I got lost in a maze of corridors and I could not find my way out. I thought, My God, this therapy is affecting me! As I was wandering around all over the hospital I had the fantasy that a nurse, or supportive nurturing woman, would take me by the hand and show me the way out. I felt completely prepubescent.

THERAPIST: So, you felt prepubescent and you wanted a woman to take you by the hand and show you the way out!

PATIENT: Yes, I thought I needed a woman or nurse because they are much more understanding and supportive than the doctors, who are busy running and paying no attention to anyone around them. Yes, I felt prepubescent and I wanted a woman to help me out.

THERAPIST: Do you view doctors as being males?

PATIENT: Yes. Although I know that this is not necessarily the case.

THERAPIST: So, you view male doctors who are all busy as being unsympathetic?

PATIENT: Yes.

THERAPIST: Does that include me too, who after all was responsible for all your anxiety when we were discussing your sexuality with your seductive father last week?

PATIENT: Yup.

THERAPIST: So, can we hear your feelings about my being unsympathetic like these other doctors? Now, we know that last week you viewed me as being like your grandfather so as to avoid seeing me being as your father, although this had been the case the previous session.

PATIENT: Well, I was running away from someone who made me anxious to a woman who could be helpful to me.

THERAPIST: Is this woman, this nurse, a mother figure?

PATIENT: Well—yes

THERAPIST: So, after a discussion about sexuality with me, who in the past you had seen as having certain features of your grandfather and your father—

PATIENT (interrupting): Yes, because I viewed you as having a different lifestyle from my own—a lifestyle like my father's or my grandfather's.

THERAPIST: So, if we pull this whole thing togeher we have the following situation: In last week's session you were very anxious as we discussed sexuality in reference to your father, who was supposed to have been very seductive, and you were aghast when your friend commented on it. As a result of this discussion, and to avoid it, you started viewing me like your grandfather, who is dead and whose lifestyle I share. Now, in reality, I am closer to your father's age, rather than your grandfather's age. As the hour was coming to an end you wanted to run away. Now, what we didn't know then that we know now is that after you left, you got lost in the hospital corridors feeling prepubescent and having the fantasy that a nurse—a woman, a mother figure—would take you by the hand and show you the way out of the hospital labyrinth, where the doctors, whom you view as being male, were too busy to pay attention to you. Furthermore, we equated that you had the same feelings for me, whom you viewed as responsible for your anxiety because of the subject of sexuality.

PATIENT: Yes.

THERAPIST: So, what we see is a shift from the sexual feelings which you expressed for your father to a wish for your mother to take you by the hand and help you out. So, are you feeling prepubescent, going to your mother for support in order to avoid competing with her, which you have been doing all along in order to make peace with her? Are you going to your mother saying, "Mommy, I don't want to compete with you and defeat you even in this sexual area. I am a little girl, a little, little prepubescent girl, so there is no sexual competition between us. Take my hand and help me out"?

PATIENT: Well, yes! This is the case.

In this way, the therapist, using a past-transference link, was able to utilize it effectively in making an important interpretation to the patient. Furthermore, it should be kept in mind that the patient was regressing with a prepubescent fantasy in an effort to avoid competing with her mother, but in reality she was dressed like a grown-up, sexual woman. Thus she was giving two different messages to her parents—a nonsexual one to her mother and a sexual one to her father-therapist.

One final example about past-transference links may also be in order.

JH, a 35-year-old artist, after the sixth session, during which he discussed his masochistic tendencies in reference to his relationship with both men and women, began the seventh as follows:

PATIENT: I have been thinking about this therapy. I had heard that it was called "anxiety-provoking" but I have not felt very much anxiety here. I had expected that it would have been more painful.

THERAPIST: This is of interest. Can we hear more about it?

PATIENT: I have visualized that this therapy was going to be like surgery. Someone whom you had treated told me you had a tendency to stick to a point like a bulldog, and that you dissected everything very systematically.

THERAPIST: You seem to be in a very medical mood today!

PATIENT: Well, you are a doctor. The other therapist whom I saw once or twice was a social worker.

THERAPIST: My being a doctor reminds you of anything?

PATIENT: Yes, my appendectomy.

THERAPIST: Now, let us hear more about all this.

PATIENT: I was seven years old. I had this pain in my belly. I remember being in the hospital. The surgeon was getting ready and told the anesthetist to go ahead. They put a mask on me and then, drop, drop, drop, the ether. I counted backwards and then I was out. That night I woke up. I was in pain. I got out of bed because I was alone and I had heard some kids playing outside of my room. I wanted to be with them. I was very lonely and I wished my father was there, but he must have been busy operating on someone else. At that point I heard someone outside of my room, so I hid in the closet. There was quite a commotion, people came in, I suppose the nurses didn't know what had happened to me. Once they found me in the closet they placed me in bed and put a net over me so as not to be able to get out of bed again. I remember I was very restless and got all tangled up by this net. I felt very sad and abandoned by everybody.

THERAPIST: So, your father was a doctor?

PATIENT: Yes.He was the one who operated one me. He removed my appendix.

THERAPIST: Oh, I see! In the same way as you wanted me to be like a surgeon, viewing this therapy like a surgery where I was supposed to dissect things very systematically, so there is a wish that I would be like your father.

PATIENT: Yes. I have thought of that before. You see, my father was very busy. Many times I wanted to be with him, but he had no time. The only occasion when he was available to me, and seemed to care, was when I was sick.

THERAPIST: So, being sick medically or psychologically gets your father's and my attention. Is that correct?

PATIENT: Well, yes. You see, when I first called to make an appointment with you I had to call several times because your line was busy. It is curious because I thought then, "Hm, he is busy like my father!"

This past-transference link in the early part of STAPP established a valuable connection between the patient's father and his therapist and was utilized effectively during his subsequent treatment.

AVOIDANCE OF PREGENITAL CHARACTEROLOGICAL ISSUES USED DEFENSIVELY BY THE PATIENT AND OF DEVELOPMENT OF TRANSFERENCE NEUROSIS

One of the key technical features of STAPP which causes it to differ greatly from other forms of brief dynamic psychotherapy as they have been used by various investigators, such as Davanloo (1978) in Montreal, Eitinger, Heiberg, and others (1975) in Oslo, Schneider (1976) and Gillieron in Lausanne, Malan (1976a) in London, and Mann (1973) in Boston, has to do with the systematic avoidance of discussion of the patient's pregenital characterological issues. The reason for this technical point has to do with the fact that the discussion of dependent needs, passive reactions, acting-out tendencies, etc., prolongs the treatment unnecessarily.

It should be remembered that STAPP patients have been evaluated thoroughly and have been found to be good candidates because they do *not* possess serious pregenital characterological problems. If such issues do surface during the therapy, it must be because the patient is using them defensively to avoid talking about the focal Oedipal issues which give rise to anxiety. It is the task of the therapist under those conditions to bring the patient back on the right focus and to disregard these defensive maneuvers on his part, which usually take the form of exaggerated castration fears or pseudohomosexual desires.

Another reason why the therapist should avoid discussion of pregenital characterological issues has to do with the development of the transference neurosis. Every effort should be made by the therapist to avoid the onset of a transference neurosis because, once it appears, it leads to an impasse. Characterological issues of a pregenital nature signal the impending development of a transference neurosis, and this is why they are bypassed. If, on the other hand, the therapist starts paying attention to such issues because he is insecure about his original evaluation of the patient's problem, then he encourages the patient to go on talking, for example, about his dependent needs, instead of his incestuous heterosexual longings which make him anxious.

Other investigators claim that they are not worried so much about the development of a transference neurosis. I, on the other hand, think that because we do not use free association and thus do not have access to all the patients' fantasies, if the transference neurosis were allowed to take place in a once-a-week face-to-face interaction, we would be unable to analyze it and the therapy would bog down. Thus every effort should be made to help the patients resolve their difficulties quickly before its onset.

Here is an example of the avoidance of pregenital characterological issues used defensively by a 23-year-old female secretary who had a strong and very sexualized attachment for her grandfather, who lived with her and her mother while she was growing up. Her own father had died during World War II, when she was an infant. By the fifth session, several therapist–parent connections had already been made. It was following that interview that the therapist had to cancel the appointment for the sixth session. He had already mentioned this cancellation to the patient. During that session, however, she chose to talk extensively about her positive transference feelings for him. She described her therapy in glowing terms. She mentioned how much she enjoyed dressing up in her best clothes to please her therapist, and how she liked to look attractive. The patient left that interview feeling very good.

Two weeks later, she returned looking somewhat unkempt, wearing a pair of old dungarees. Her hair was pulled back and was not very well combed, which gave her a dejected expression. She was frowning as she walked slowly in and flopped on her chair. She was silent at first, and when she started to talk, she said that she felt tired and sick. The therapist listened to her for a while, and then he pointed out to her the difference in her appearance between the two sessions:

PATIENT: I am not feeling very well today, as I have told you already. I feel sick. I want you to do the talking for a while. I want something soothing today. After all, it's partly your fault that I'm feeling the way I do today. I'm achy, I have—

THERAPIST (*interrupting*): And why is it my fault?

PATIENT: Because you did not make an offer to give me another appointment after you canceled the one last week.

THERAPIST: We discussed all this before.

PATIENT: Yes, I know, but you never offered to make up the time.

THERAPIST: If you wanted another appointment, why didn't you ask for one?

PATIENT: You canceled it, so it was up to you to give me another one.

THERAPIST: What's going on today?

PATIENT: I told you that I wanted to be soothed.

THERAPIST: I'm not going to soothe you, and you know better than that. Now, stop feeling sorry· for yourself and let's get back to work.

PATIENT (*sarcastic*): I don't feel like being self-inquisitive today.

THERAPIST: So, you are self-destructive today. Having had no hour last week, which you blame on me, now you are determined to waste this hour so as to be even with me. Now, what about all this appointment controversy?

PATIENT: I told you that I wanted you to offer me another appointment.

THERAPIST: I know that. I also said that you could have asked for one if you wanted to. You are entitled to ask for what you want, in a mature way, but you are not entitled to act like a little spoiled child in here, because this is what we try to help you understand and overcome. Now, let me clarify something which I am sure you know only too well. I deal with you as a grown-up person, not as a child, and furthermore, I am not here to play soothing games. Now, are you going to settle down and get to work, which you are perfectly capable of performing, as you have already demonstrated, or not?

PATIENT: It's always like this whenever I make an effort to straighten things out. I get kicked in the teeth. I remember once when my grandfather said that he would have liked me to get an A in geography because it was his favorite subject. So I worked and worked and on my next report card I got an A. I was very proud and when I got home, I rushed up to my grandfather's room to show him my report card, but to my great disappointment he didn't even look at it. He was busy packing his suitcase to go on a business trip. He said, "Not now, honey, can't you see I'm busy?" I ran out of his room. I locked myself in the bathroom and I cried and cried. He soon realized that my feelings were hurt and he came pleading with me to come out, but I didn't. I kept on thinking, "All that work for nothing!"

THERAPIST: You are dead wrong! You got an A in geography, you learned something about that subject. These were benefits which you got for *yourself*. The one thing you did not get was the praise you expected from your grandfather. I can understand your disappointment, but it should be a lesson to you. If you depend on others instead of relying on yourself, then you get hurt. Now, what interests me is that we have the exact parallel of this episode with your grandfather right here in reference to the appointment with me.

PATIENT: Hmmm . . . .

THERAPIST: Now, it is not surprising that you view me as your grandfather, which we have already discussed. It is not surprising, therefore, that you're experiencing here the same feelings of being sorry for yourself you experienced at that time. There are two ways, however, of looking at your reaction to all this. The first one is this "poor me" passive and dependent maladaptive attitude, all for the sake of another person, which results from your own angry feelings. The second is a better way of handling things, and it has to do with taking matters into your hands and standing on your own two feet. It is this healthier attitude that I am trying to reinforce because it is this desire of yours which motivated you to come to the clinic. Isn't this true?

PATIENT: Yes, it is.

THERAPIST: Okay, then. Furthermore, your remembering this episode about your report card was evidence of your determination to get better. I suspect that when you realized I was not going to go along with your neurotic ways, you decided that it was time to start working again.

The therapist clearly takes a strong stand against the patient's demands to be soothed. He also does not let her go on with the description of her symptoms but quickly deals with her projection onto him. It is his fault, she says, for the way she feels. By rejecting this assumption, by persisting in challenging her defensive maneuvers, by avoiding involvement in her dependent needs, he encourages her to resume their therapeutic work. He is finally rewarded by some interesting associations on her part which tend to solidify their therapeutic link.

It should not be concluded from this discussion, however, that the therapist is always anxiety-provoking and that he never supports the patient. Far from it. One indeed suggests, encourages and reinforces the patient's efforts to face anxiety, to bring up painful associations, and to arrive at unpleasant realizations. When the therapist observes that the patient is making an effort to understand himself and to resolve his difficulties but seems to have a hard time in the process, he does everything he can to support him.

NEW LEARNING AND PROBLEM SOLVING BY THE PATIENT, AND THE THERAPIST'S INTERPRETATIONS

The importance of the role played by learning in psychotherapy has always been emphasized by psychologists, while the contributors of learning theory have by and large been ignored by the psychoanalysts (Porter, 1968). That new learning was taking place during the course of short-term psychotherapy was one of the first findings which we discovered from our follow-up interviews (Sifneos, 1972). The description of the treatment as a "new learning experience," as a "course tailor-made" for the patient, or as a "problem-solving device" impressed us greatly because it pointed to the cognitive component, and because it seemed to be as important as the affective element which up to that time had been viewed as playing the dominant role in the patient's successful outcome. The ability to verbalize the psychodynamics, and to emphasize that self-understanding has developed during the therapy, provides the patient with a novel way to learn to look into himself, and helps in the resolution of his problem. Because of this, we decided that we should pay special attention to the investigation of these cognitive understandings.

It is obvious, however, that such new learning and problem solving cannot take place without the therapist's repeated interpretations. After all, the patient has had all these various ingredients available to him for a long time, yet he has been unable to solve his psychological difficulties. If he has managed to succeed during the therapy, it must be because of the work that was done with the therapist.

In the same way as with confrontation and clarification, interpretation must be timed properly and must be based on solid evidence of details provided by the patient. The best way to make such interpretations is for the therapist to summarize periodically the progress which has been made up to that time by recapitulating the material dealing with transference as well as with the therapist–parent connections. These interpretations constitute a novel explanation of the patient's difficulties, and they carry with them potential solutions which the patient had not thought of before. Despite the fact that at times they may seem unpalatable and painful, their originality becomes striking and their potential advantages begin to have an impact.

The patient soon starts to identify with the therapist and imitates the way he goes about analyzing the information. This type of identification with the therapist and his interpretations becomes a great asset to the patient because he is excited not only by the prospects of new ways to understand his problem but also by the potential which such insights may have for him in other situations. The patient is now able to have tangible evidence that he can indeed solve his psychological problems. For example, a young man with a neurotic pattern of dealing with women has learned that this attitude resulted from his earlier relation with his mother; when he is able to start interacting with his new girlfriend in a very different manner, his enthusiasm has no limits. He realizes quickly that his old ways of handling his problems were outmoded; the new patterns of behavior offer him far better opportunities for success. No wonder, then, that he is willing to utilize what he has learned to solve not only his current problem but also other problems which he may encounter in his life, long after the therapy has come to an end.

One cannot overemphasize the importance of preparing the ground very carefully before the therapist makes an interpretation. He must review his notes, and preferably utilize certain key words which the patient has used to describe a specific event, a special memory, or a vivid fantasy. His observations about the patient's behavior must be clearly summarized in his mind and a distinct problem-solving interpretation must be prepared, with no speculative aspects attached to it. There should be no doubts in the therapist's mind about its relevance. He must then proceed to present his facts clearly and forcibly, using language as simple as possible, free of any jargon. He must pursue his presentation almost stubbornly, even in the face of resistance from the patient, which at times can be fierce. Even if he has to talk most of the time during the interview, he should constantly challenge the patient to reinterpret in a different way the facts which are presented to him, and if the patient is unable to do so, he should urge him to accept the therapist's interpretation because it is based on true observations. He should continue making his point and repeat it several times until he is finally able to obtain the full agreement and cooperation of the patient, until he is absolutely sure that the patient has a clear understanding of his own dynamics.

As soon as this has been accomplished, the patient will start realizing the implications of this novel way of understanding himself in terms of the valuable possibilities which are opened to him to free himself from his neurotic difficulties. He will then start seeing the light at the end of the tunnel!

It should not be forgotten that problem solving usually is followed by a release of considerable positive affect.

McGuire has emphasized the importance of instruction of conflict identifications and resolutions so as to learn to use these techniques effectively under similar clinical circumstances. He also thought that structuring information and putting it in a sequence which is most natural for the patient helps greatly in the problem-solving process (McGuire, 1970).

Problem solving has been repeatedly mentioned by our patients as having been a crucial aspect of their STAPP, helping them to solve psychological problems long after their treatment has come to an end. Thus it can be pointed out that technical factors play an important role in making psychotherapy effective, contrary to the belief by some investigators that nonspecific factors such as empathy and support are the only effective therapeutic components of psychotherapy.

Thus the height of the treatment has been reached! Let us now see how one of our male STAPP patients was able to deal with his problems at this phase of his treatment, how his therapist effectively interpreted his psychodynamics to him, and how this joint venture produced a resolution of his Oedipal psychological problem.

CHAPTER 9

The Height of the
Therapy: A Case Example

All the technical features of STAPP discussed in previous chapters will be demonstrated in the following case example of the height of the treatment, with a typical candidate.*

The patient was a 32-year-old man who came to the clinic because of the sudden onset of obsessive-compulsive symptoms during his honeymoon. It appeared that as his wife was opening a wedding present, she seemed to have strewn the wrappings all over the floor of their hotel room. At that point the patient experienced intense anger at his wife, but soon after he started very meticulously to pick up the papers off the floor. Ever since then he had the urge to pick up paper or pieces of litter from the floor or from the street so as to make sure that everything was perfectly clean. Soon afterward he started to be obsessed by the thought that he was in some way responsible for his father's death. He realized the absurdity of these thoughts and acts but had difficulty in stopping them.

The patient was a tall, thin, attractive man. He was very bright, and was very successful as a young professor of classics in a local university. He had very good relations with various members of his family as a child, and had many good friends during his adoles-

---

* A brief description of this patient's psychotherapy appeared in Sifneos (1966) and Sifneos (1972, pp. 109–113).

cence and his adult life. He interacted very well with the evaluators during their interviews.

Soon after the sudden death of his father, which occurred six months before he came for treatment, he met his future wife. They were married four months later.

His motivation to understand the cause of his psychological difficulties was very high. Thus it was thought that he fulfilled all the selection criteria for STAPP; furthermore, there was an Oedipal focus that could be established easily. He was very attached to his mother and older sister. His relations with his father had also been very good, but at times there were competitive feelings between them in sports as well as when they discussed religious matters. His father was a very devout Catholic and had also wanted his son to be religious, but the patient seemed to have been uninterested in the church, and hated to attend mass on Sundays with his father. Confession and communion were what annoyed him most. He thought that his own ideas should be kept private, and he felt very angry at being judged as sinful or being absolved of any fictitious sins.

The contract with the patient was agreed upon, and he was very eager to start his psychotherapy.

The critera for improvement which we specified involved the disappearance of his obsessive-compulsive symptoms, the understanding of his relationship with his father, and the lack of displacing his anger from his father onto his wife. One would also expect a diminution of the intensity of his anger.

The first few interviews were essentially uneventful. The patient talked a great deal about his good relations with women in general, and his sister and mother in particular. As the therapy went on, however, he started to be evasive and was confronted about it by the therapist. He continued to avoid details and appeared to generalize. He became more and more evasive. As the therapist pressed him continuously to come to grips with his conflicts, he started to become angry. The transference feelings, however, up to that time had been predominantly positive.

He came 10 minutes late for his ninth interview and the following exchange took place after the patient was silent for a while:

THERAPIST: You are silent today.
PATIENT (*angrily*): You are blaming me for being late?

THERAPIST: You seem to be projecting your feelings onto me. I pointed to your silence, not to your being late. Are the two connected?

PATIENT: I'm sorry. I didn't mean to yell at you. (*He was again silent for a while, then suddenly he said*): An entirely irrelevant episode from my childhood seems to have crossed my mind.

THERAPIST: Go on. (*Although the therapist wants to revert to the transference exchange, he is intrigued by the "irrelevant episode" and decides to pursue his inquiry about it.*)

PATIENT: I remember going fishing with my father. It was one of the best things that we did together. What went through my mind was an episode when I was twelve, when I accidentally dropped my fishing rod in the lake. I went after it to retrieve it and almost overturned our canoe. My father was very mad. He said, "You're always so careful! How could you be so careless? I could have drowned."

THERAPIST: Did he say, "*I* could have drowned" or "*We* could have drowned"?

PATIENT: No. I remember very clearly that he said "I."

THERAPIST: So, the implication is that you would have been saved?

PATIENT: I guess so. No, I don't know. He thought only of himself.

THERAPIST: Well, what about it then?

PATIENT: I felt very angry at my dad. I remember it clearly, but I'm not sure if it was because he was selfish or because he criticized me.

THERAPIST: He was justified in criticizing you.

PATIENT (*irritably*): Yes, I know, but it didn't have to be in that tone! Then I remember thinking, "How can my dad be so sloppy and leave his desk in such a mess?" (*He was again silent.*) Maybe he should have drowned. . . .

THERAPIST: What are you thinking about right now?

PATIENT: You also have all these sheets of paper on your desk.

THERAPIST: So, there's a connection between your father and me. (*From the evidence given to him by the patient, the therapist takes the opportunity to make a therapist–parent connection.*)

PATIENT: Yes, because I feel the same irritation at you as I did about my father. You see, Dad didn't give up. After we returned from the fishing trip, he called me into his study and kept talking to me about safety. He gave me a lecture. He said, furthermore, that if I wasn't going to be careful, then he wouldn't go fishing with me anymore. I didn't care. The only thing I can remember was all that paper strewn all over his desk.

THERAPIST: Like those papers that you were picking up off the floor of your hotel room during your honeymoon?

PATIENT: That's very interesting . . . (*Then, with a smile on his face, he said irrelevantly*): You have a cute secretary.

THERAPIST: Hmm . . . tell me about it.

PATIENT: She's friendly, has a nice figure, and is a blonde. I like blondes.

THERAPIST: I see.

PATIENT: She reminds me of an ex-girlfriend of mine. (*He went on to give many details about his relations with women before he was married. He seemed to have been very successful with women. Most of the rest of the interview was spent on reminiscences.*)

THERAPIST: Can we get back to my secretary, to the papers on my desk, on your father's desk, on the floor of your hotel room, to the fishing episode, and to your being late?

PATIENT: Well, you seem to have summarized the whole hour.

Indeed this was the case. The therapist would have done better if he had picked one of these issues to concentrate on. He had an embarrassment of riches and then failed to take advantage of any one of them. This was a mistake. The hour ended at that point.

One of the important tasks facing the STAPP therapist has to do with making short-term predictions between sessions after he has reviewed his notes.

SHORT-TERM PREDICTIONS BETWEEN SESSIONS, AND NOTE TAKING

The session which was summarized by the therapist can be viewed as a typical hour at the height of STAPP. The patient is working hard. Despite the negative transference feelings which appear early, the therapeutic alliance is very strong and the patient's motivation to understand himself helps him to cooperate with the therapist. Thus it is interesting to see that the patient is able to recall that important fishing episode from the past, which is clearly associated with his competitive feelings with his father and thereby gives the therapist an opportunity to make the important parent-transference link.

At this point the therapist must prepare himself for the following session. He must question what the patient's reaction will be to the preceding hour. Next time, will he bring more material from the past as he has done in reference to the fishing episode, or will his transference feelings in reference to the remark about the therapist's secretary get in his way? For example, will the patient attempt to retreat from experiencing anger for the therapist because it is too difficult to handle? Will he suppress these feelings or will he act them out in one way or other? If so, what kind of acting out should one expect the patient to perform? Will he again be late for his session? Will he show up at all? Or call to cancel his appointment, giving some kind of excuse? Of course, the acting-out could take the focus of some kind of fight with his wife, or with someone at work. Finally, will there be an aggravation of the patient's symptomatology?

All these questions must be considered by the therapist, who must prepare himself for any eventuality which is likely to take place so as not to be caught by surprise. One of the best ways to do this is for the therapist to review his notes carefully in order not to miss any important piece of information which he may have disregarded. Thus good note taking is, in my opinion, a *sine qua non* for STAPP. I have always advocated taking written notes during the interview and have done so without its interfering in any way with the interaction between therapist and patient. Furthermore, this is true from my observations of those whom I have supervised who were also willing to take written notes.

Written note taking offers the therapist the invaluable advantage of having the exact sequence of the therapeutic material without having to rely on his memory, good as it may be. If one takes notes after the end of the hour, there is a tendency to remember those aspects discussed toward the latter part of the interview, while the earlier happenings of the session may become confused.

Another advantage has to do with taking down certain statements of the patient verbatim, and describing his reactions following an anxiety-provoking confrontation or interpretation. When the therapist repeats the patient's exact words to him, or is able to present him with a reaction which he may not have been aware of, or was willing to avoid, to suppress, or to bypass, the impact of such an interpretation can be much more effective.

As a result of the review of his notes, the therapist predicted that the patient's reaction to the hour would take a pattern similar to what had happened before, namely, that he was again going to act out by coming late for his interview. Thus the negative transference feelings would have to be clarified during the forthcoming hour.

Tenth Interview

The patient was 15 minutes late for his appointment. He went on as follows:

PATIENT: My compulsion to pick up papers was much worse this week.

It is obvious that the therapist had underestimated the patient's regressive pattern, which took the form of an aggravation of his symptoms, but was right that some sort of acting-out would take place. Therefore, he was ready to deal with the acting-out, while deciding that further pursuit of the symptomatic complaints should be bypassed because, if they were discussed, they would tend to encourage the patient to retreat into his complaints about his symptoms and bring about some of his more regressive pregenital characterological issues (which should always be avoided as much as possible).

THERAPIST: But you are also late, as you were last week.
PATIENT: I'm sorry about that, but it was because of my symptoms. I waste so much time on them I'm not getting any better. In fact, I'm getting worse. I started to have doubts about this therapy, yet I know that such thoughts are destructive. I seem to be helpless. I can't stop this self-defeating attitude, yet I do want to understand myself. (*He was silent for a while and then he went on*): This was a bad week. All these compulsions of mine drove me mad. I cleared up my desk four times yesterday. It's ridiculous, I know, but I couldn't stop myself. (*He went on for a while longer describing his symptoms.*)

THERAPIST: It seems to me that you want to convey the impression that you are the victim. You feel sorry for yourself, yet you don't want to ask the obvious question, whether clearing your desk four times is directly connected with your father's and my desk, as we talked about last week.

PATIENT (*becoming visibly pale*): I have the urge to empty the contents of the wastebasket on your desk. This is irrelevant I know, but by God, I'd very much like to do it.

THERAPIST: There we go again! Your honeymoon all over again, but in reverse. (*The therapist was referring to the onset of the patient's symptoms during his honeymoon when he had the urge to pick up the wrappings of his wife's wedding gift off the floor.*)

PATIENT: Oh, no, it's rather the thought that I was responsible for my father's death that makes me feel so upset. This thought has been preoccupying me lately. It's a terrible thought. I feel so guilty. (*His hands started to shake.*)

THERAPIST: As you know, you have similar feelings for your father and for me, and last week—

PATIENT: Drop dead! (*He said this defiantly, then he blushed and added*): Then I can sleep with your secretary.

THERAPIST: Hm! So, if I die, it will become easier for you to take away my secretary, whom you find so attractive. Did you also want to take your mother away from your father, and is that why you wished both of us dead? (*This confrontation had an immediate effect.*)

PATIENT (*becoming visibly relaxed and laughing*): Oh, this is silly!

THERAPIST: Oh, is it, eh? If so, why are you so frightened and guilty about this thought that you are responsible for your father's death? Why do you blush and your hands shake? Are all your obsessions and compulsions a way to expiate your crime, the crime of wanting your father to die, in the same way as you wished me dead? Yet now you want to avoid all this feeling by calling it silly. This is not a very brave way of dealing with your competitors. Why can't you compete on a one-to-one basis, openly and freely? Why do you have to go underground? If you are attracted to my secretary, you have to kill me off, so it would be easier for you to pursue your conquest, but you pay a huge price for this neurotic wish. Your death wishes for your father and for me serve no purpose except to increase your guilt. It's much better to have the

courage to look at all this straight in the eye. Let's try to understand what is going on, not avoid it.

PATIENT: The strange thing is that I feel better.

The patient spent the rest of the hour reminiscing about the
good times that he had with his father. The therapist let him talk
because he felt that he was trying indirectly to emphasize that,
despite his death wishes, he was fond of both his father and the
therapist.

THERAPIST: I think from what you say that you want to communicate that you loved your father despite your death wishes
for him. I know you did. It is precisely because you did love your
father that you experienced such intensive guilt feelings. I think
that you are ready to try to solve this problem. The time is up for
today, but let's try again next week.

The technical aspects of STAPP which have already been described are evident during this session. The therapist avoided getting involved in the pregenital characterological defensive features,
the patient's self-pity. Although it could be argued that he could
have done it earlier, the therapist does manage to get the patient to
deal with what had been discussed during the previous sessions.
He is immediately rewarded by a series of interesting associations:
first, the wish to empty the contents of the watebasket all over the
therapist's desk; second, the association about the fears of being
responsible for his father's death; finally, the death wish for the
therapist and the desire to sleep with his secretary. Thus it is clear
that, as a result of the parent-transference connection, the patient's
feelings for his father are openly transferred onto the therapist during the interview. The therapist's task is clear for the next hour. He
must proceed to clarify the Oedipal focus and to help the patient
find a different, more appropriate, and more adaptive solution to
his neurotic problem.

Eleventh Interview

The patient was early for this session.

PATIENT: I had an interesting dream last night. I was on a safari
with one of my old girlfriends, when suddenly out of the bush

jumped a huge ostrich. It was more like a giraffe full of mul-
ticolored feathers. Its face had a fierce expression on it, then it
started to chase me. I was terrified, but I didn't want to show it. I
wanted to kill the damned thing. I thought despite my fear that if
I could shoot it down, Pat (*his girlfriend*) would be impressed with
me. I suddenly noticed that I was holding a gun. I lifted it and
aimed straight at it, but when I pulled the trigger, it wouldn't
fire. I woke up in a cold sweat. I was drenched!

THERAPIST: What are your associations to your dream?

PATIENT: I don't know. I thought it was an important dream, and I
wanted to tell you about it, but as soon as you asked me, very
little seems to come to my mind.

THERAPIST: So, you block, but it won't do you any good. Don't try
to run away. What are your associations to this important dream?

PATIENT (*hesitating*): Nothing directly in reference to the dream.

THERAPIST: What comes to mind? Go on.

PATIENT: I remembered an episode when I was young . . . (hesitating).

THERAPIST: Go ahead, carry on.

PATIENT: I remembered once when Julie, my older sister, was taking
a shower, I tried to peek through the keyhole. I didn't do it with
anyone else, but I did it when Julie was taking her shower. I was
vaguely aware that I wasn't supposed to be doing what I was
doing.

THERAPIST: How old were you?

PATIENT: Oh, about six.

THERAPIST: How old was Julie?

PATIENT: Julie must have been . . . let's see . . . about fourteen or
so. . . . You see, Dad liked Julie very much. I think she was his
favorite. Come to think of it, my father liked women very much.
Julie was very well developed, you know, she had very well-
developed breasts, but what I remember most about those times
. . . I mean, when I was looking through the keyhole, was her
pubic hair.

He went on and talked in some detail about various experiences with his older sister as well as his younger sister. He referred
to his sisters and his mother as his "father's women." Then, as if
remembering what he had blocked, he said that he remembered

another episode, but at the same time he again became shaky and hesitating:

THERAPIST: Don't block. What did you remember?

PATIENT: I remember one time when my father had returned from a fishing trip. He had gone by himself and had caught several large rainbow trout. He was very proud of his success. I remember that he called me into the kitchen to show them to me. I was very excited. I ran down and there on the kitchen table were all the fish, but what struck my attention (*shivering*) . . . well, there was a large one without a head. It had been decapitated accidentally. (*He looked very uncomfortable.*) Even now I shudder at the thought.

THERAPIST: What is the thought?

PATIENT: That my father could be very cruel. If he could do what he did to that poor fish . . .

THERAPIST: But why does that make *you* anxious?

PATIENT: If he could do it to the fish, he could do it to me.

THERAPIST: For peeping through the keyhole at one of "his women."

PATIENT (*taken aback*): That's amazing! . . . (*visibly more relaxed*) You know, the strange thing is that my father was never very punitive. In actuality, he was very kind. A very benign sort of a person, he was—

THERAPIST: I think this reality created more problems for you. We know that you loved your father. We know that he was a "benign sort of a person." We also know that he liked "his women"— Julie, your mother, your younger sister.

PATIENT: Yes, that's all very true.

THERAPIST: I think that you have exaggerated your father's potential punishment of you in this episode of the "castrated trout." You make him look like an ogre, like an executioner, who cut heads off when he is angry and when he wants to retaliate against people who challenge his authority and who have an interest in Julie. In reality, however, your father is kind. Now, tell me, why didn't your gun fire in your dream?

The patient was silent. It was the end of the hour.

In terms of the dynamics of the case, I think that the patient's castration anxiety and the defense mechanisms which he used to deal with it are quite obvious. In the same way as one does in psychoanalysis, the dream is utilized during STAPP to tie the material from the previous interview to the present one, although in the case of STAPP the two sessions are one week apart.

It will be remembered that at the end of the tenth interview the patient was challenged to compete openly with the therapist—as a father substitute—and not to run away. It is obvious that this was too much for the patient to be expected to do at this stage of the therapy, so he tried to deal with this situation somewhat less directly. The dream offered a perfect compromise. If he became impotent, and his gun would not fire, then he would not be punished with "decapitation." This interesting association brought into the open his sexual curiosity for one of his father's "women," Julie, and his fear of punishment for it.

It is obvious that the regressive solution of his dilemma is a neurotic one. The therapist must therefore encourage him to face his fears and not to retreat to a castrated state, which is represented by his being the victim, with neurotic obsessive-compulsive symptoms, feeling sorry for himself. Thus, he must encourage the patient to find a more mature resolution of his Oedipal struggle, and this is what he is prepared to do during the following session.

Twelfth Interview

The patient again was on time.

PATIENT: Both the episode about the rainbow trout and the dream were very much on my mind during the past week, but I felt better and my compulsions decreased considerably.

THERAPIST: I'm glad to hear it, but don't forget the episode with your sister Julie, her shower, and your sexual curiosity for your "father's woman"!

PATIENT (cooperatively): And don't forget my wanting to impress my girlfriend in the dream.

THERAPIST: Indeed, as well as your interest for my secretary!

PATIENT: Hm . . .

THERAPIST: Generally speaking, you haven't talked very much up to now about your relations with women during your adolescence. Can we hear something about them?

The patient talked about his success with women. It was as if a
green light had been turned on. He went on relating with great relish his sexual experiences, but the one thing which seemed to
emerge quite clearly was his interest in women who were engaged,
married, or in one way or another unavailable. He also had a great
urge to flirt with the girlfriends of his close friends.

PATIENT: I remember when there was that dinner celebrating Jim's
engagement. He was my college roommate, to whom I was very
much attached. During that whole dinner, I felt an overwhelming
desire for his fiancée, although.I had a date with Elaine, who was
a very attractive young woman. It was like a compulsion to have
Wendy, Jim's fiancée, be interested in me. I knew that he was
very jealous, but somehow I couldn't resist the temptation. I also
knew that Wendy liked me, but I was determined to have her be
attracted to me. During dinner she was sitting on my left and Jim
sat next to her on her left. I talked to Wendy throughout dinner,
and I saw to it that her glass was always full of wine. I also told
her a lot of dirty jokes. She laughed and laughed. Then I accidentally touched her knee and suddenly felt an overwhelming urge to
caress her thigh. I knew it was dangerous but I felt compelled to
do it.
THERAPIST: There are a lot of compulsions today!
PATIENT: Yes, indeed!
THERAPIST: Go on.
PATIENT: Well! (*He continued with great enthusiasm, almost as if drunk
with excitement*): I just decided that I had to risk it to see what she
was going to do. I put my hand on Wendy's left knee and left it
there. I was amazed because I expected her to push my hand off,
but she didn't. I was elated (*with a big smile on his face*), so I got
bolder and I started to caress her thigh. She seemed to enjoy it all.
I was tempted to raise my hand up to her pubic area, but it would
have been a bit difficult to do and—
THERAPIST (*interrupting*): You seem to enjoy greatly talking about all
this, in contrast to last week's hour when you were so anxious.
Tell me, are you saying all this to impress me? You have a trium-
phant smile on your face. You see, Wendy is not my secretary.
The question is, why did you have to sneak?
PATIENT (*irritably*): What do you mean "sneak"?
THERAPIST: Exactly that. If you wanted to seduce Wendy, you

should have had the courage to do it openly and honestly. You should have told your roommate that you were attracted to her. You should have told your own date the same thing. You shouldn't have been trying to deceive them by playing all these childish games under the table.

PATIENT (*looking very angry*): Damn you!

THERAPIST: You are very angry, of course, because it is the truth and you don't like it. You know, I hope, that it is the truth. You have tried to solve the problem of being attracted to your sister, to Wendy, and to my secretary by trying to deceive your father, Jim, and me. You peek through the keyhole, you go under the table, you wish I'd drop dead, so as to get what you want. You put on this weak, "poor me" cover-up. You develop neurotic compulsions in order to cover up your desires. As I have already told you, be honest with yourself and with all of us. I know that you are capable of doing it. All these things have happened in the past. We must now, right here, try to understand why your marriage stirred all this up. Do you know why?

PATIENT (*shaking his head, but looking subdued*): No.

THERAPIST: Do you want to find out?

PATIENT (*with emphasis*): Yes, I do. (*His anger seemed to have vanished.*)

THERAPIST: Okay, then, let's try to figure all this out. You haven't told me very much about your wife except when you described that episode about the wedding present. What does your wife look like?

PATIENT: She's tall. She has blue eyes. She has a very nice figure, but she's prematurely gray.

THERAPIST: Whom does she remind you of?

PATIENT: Well, Julie is also tall and has blue eyes.

THERAPIST: Julie, eh? . . . and does she also have gray hair?

PATIENT: No, Julie doesn't.

THERAPIST: Who does?

PATIENT: (*hesitating*): Well, Mom does.

THERAPIST: Oh, I see. So she is a composite of Julie and your mother. Tell me, what would your father think if he knew about all this?

PATIENT: I never thought of it this way . . . . It's amazing, by God . . . I remember when I was young that I was happiest when my mother gave her dinner parties.

THERAPIST: What do you mean "her dinner parties"?

PATIENT: You see, my father didn't like dinner parties. As you know, he liked to go fishing or hunting and at times would be away for two or three days. During these absences my mother would have her dinner parties. They were glorious events. Mother was a good cook, and she would prepare all those special dishes. She also loved wine and would choose the various bottles of wine to go with each dish. I was allowed to open the bottles and take them to the dining room. When the guests arrived, my mother would let me serve the hors d'oeuvres. She was always beautifully dressed, and so was Julie, who was always surrounded by admirers, but I always sat next to her.

THERAPIST: Just like sitting next to Wendy?

PATIENT: By God, that's fantastic! I never thought of it. It's amazing! (*He went on reminiscing about his mother's parties. When the hour was approaching the end, the therapist went on as follows*):

THERAPIST: Well, all the ingredients are here. Summing up what we have learned today, it seems to me that you married someone who had many of the attributes of your mother and your older sister, Julie. On your honeymoon this realization, which was only partially conscious, brought you back to the old times when you had desires for your "father's women" and competed with him, yet you also feared his punishment. Thus you developed your symptoms, your obsessions and compulsions which made you appear the victim, a castrated victim at that. But it was a way to appease your father, whose punishment you were terrified of as we saw so clearly in the trout episode. Your wishing your father dead was a way out, but, unfortunately, it didn't work out very well because it gave rise to your guilt feelings. After your father died, you started to think that you were responsible for his death because of these death wishes. The main trouble about all this was your effort to hide your sexual interests by being what I already called "deceitful," which made you feel so mad. That indeed was a neurotic way of dealing with the situation and could have created a lot of difficulties for you. For example, you could have lost your roommate, whom, as we know, you liked very much. Finally, I think we have been able to reexamine all this here. You reexperienced the old feelings of competition and anger for your father here in reference to me. We have seen here the arousal of your sexual desires for "his women" in reference to my secretary. It seems that all the pieces of the jigsaw puzzle have been put in place. The whole picture is now very clear. What do you think?

PATIENT: Indeed . . . it's just amazing!

In the next sessions, the patient's symptoms improved greatly. Therapy was terminated soon afterward. It had lasted four months, 16 interviews in all.

This case was chosen, as already mentioned, to demonstrate the technique of STAPP at its height. In addition, the fact that the patient suffered from obsessive-compulsive neurosis, which is usually considered difficult to treat, demonstrates that STAPP can produce rapidly a dramatic change even in this group of patients.

Several patients suffering from mild obsessive-compulsive disorder of a sudden onset were treated with STAPP, and the results were published in Sifneos (1966). At that time it was emphasized that the defensive pattern of these patients was unmistakably obsessive-compulsive in nature, but it seemed to be more fluid than what one encounters in the rigid structure of the classic obsessive-compulsive character. Anxiety seems to be present more often, as well as anger, as was seen in the treatment of this patient. Generally speaking, these individuals did well with STAPP.

At the time of termination, it was thought that the criteria which had been set for a successful outcome in this patient had almost been met. The symptoms had not disappeared completely but had improved greatly. It was thought that the symptoms would disappear by the time of the follow-up visit. Otherwise, however, it was obvious that the patient had a clear understanding of his relationship with his father, and of the complications which resulted from his sexual wishes for his sister and his mother. His relations with his wife improved greatly. He was not angry with her anymore.

When he was seen in a follow-up visit three years later, his symptoms had completely disappeared. The patient at that time described his therapy as an invaluable learning experience which saved his marriage.

Before leaving the subject of the "height of the therapy," there are some additional technical aspects which could be discussed briefly. These are recapitulation at times of massive resistance, support of the patient who is making progress, and education of the patient.

RECAPITULATION AT TIMES OF MASSIVE RESISTANCE

There are times, although rarely, that as a result of the clarifications and interpretations of the therapist the patient's anxiety may reach such a point when there seems to be a head-on collision between the two participants. When this is the case, it is wise for the therapist to stop insisting about the truth of his interpretations and use a technical device which usually brings about a resolution of the conflict, namely, "recapitulation." What is meant by this term is an effort on the part of the therapist to go back and review exactly how the therapy has developed up to that point, and to use preferably verbatim statements made by the patient in the past (here again the use of note taking comes to the assistance of the therapist). In addition, the therapist should ask the patient whether or not he agrees with the presentations of the facts, and encourage him to make corrections if the interpretations and explanations are viewed as being incorrect.

This usually breaks up the impasse and the disagreement comes to an end. The therapy can proceed from that point on uneventfully.

SUPPORT OF THE PATIENT WHO IS MAKING PROGRESS

It is generally believed that strict neutrality on the part of the analyst during psychoanalysis is an important technical stance for that form of therapy. In STAPP, on the other hand, although therapeutic neutrality is also advocated, it is nevertheless considered appropriate to encourage and support the patient and to urge him to carry on when it is evident that he is motivated to change and seems to be making progress and developing insight, despite his anxieties and difficulties.

MB, the patient who had problems about control issues and who has already been described as demonstrating transference issues and past–present links, seemed to be on the verge of tears on several occasions during one of her interviews. The following exchange took place between her and the therapist.

THERAPIST: You seem to have difficulty in discussing all these issues about sexuality. Now, what is it that bothers you most about all this? For example, we have seen it in reference to your feelings for your father, to your relations with your mother and other women, as well as about your own sexual development. So, which one of all these is most troublesome to you?

PATIENT: Well, it seems that it touches the most inner core of my self. What was my sexuality as a child? It hits to the quick. (*becoming teary*)

THERAPIST: Yes, I know this is all very difficult, but what is important is that you have the courage to confront these issues rather than to avoid them. As you know, although blocking or denying them may help temporarily, they don't solve the problem. It is like shoving things under the rug in the hope that they will disappear. Unfortunately, the bulge remains and doesn't go away. I think you are able to look at some of those frightening issues in a different way and you must go on. What do you think?

PATIENT: I guess so. Yes, I feel I must go on with all this stuff.

Although the therapist was not actively reassuring the patient, and he was urging her to continue her quest, nevertheless, he was rewarding her and reinforcing her efforts at self-understanding.

EDUCATION OF THE PATIENT

A didactic component of the patient may be a unique feature of STAPP which at times has shocked other workers in the field because it is viewed as being so unorthodox. Learning anew to problem-solve, as has already been mentioned, and developing new attitudes are actively encouraged by the therapist in order to foster the development of insight.

Thus the ability of the patient to understand the patterns of his defense mechanisms in dealing with a specific—and in the case of STAPP, Oedipal—conflict helps to set up a learning pattern for resolving problems that can be used effectively throughout the therapy and subsequently after its termination by the patient.

CHAPTER 10

The Last Phase of STAPP: An Example of a Typical Interview

The male patient whose fourth STAPP interview was described in Chapter 7 continued working hard during his therapy. Although the transference had been positive and had been dealt with appropriately by pointing out the parent-transference connections, the patient managed to avoid bringing up some of the antagonistic and angry feelings which he felt for his father. Here is a fragment of the eighth interview:

PATIENT: During the last week I remembered an episode, when I was young, which I think was significant in reference to my feelings for my mother that we were talking about. My mother was very much interested in music and insisted on my learning how to play the piano. She also supervised my practicing. On one occasion I had to play a Beethoven sonata at one of my piano teacher's periodic concerts. These took place once a year for the benefit of the parents of his students. It was the first time that I was chosen to play. My mother was thrilled, but she was after me all week to practice. The day before the concert my mother made me practice for two hours. She was so demanding and insisted that I should practice more after dinner. I was mad but I didn't say anything. I was exhausted.

THERAPIST: That reaction of yours is very familiar, isn't it?

PATIENT: You mean my reactions to my wife's angry demands, which we've talked about?

THERAPIST: Yes.

PATIENT: That's true, but what followed was of interest. You see, my father interfered and told my mother to leave me alone. She was mad at him and told him off. And you know what? My father gave up. He said to me, "Your mother wants you to practice, so you must practice."

THERAPIST: How did you feel?

PATIENT: I felt mad, but I started to argue with him. I would ask him questions, and when he replied I asked him more questions. I tried to trap him to make him admit that he was weak. I pretended to be very calm, however. My mother was amused by this discussion. She said that I sounded like a "prosecuting attorney." I was pleased by this remark.

THERAPIST: So you displaced on your poor, weak father the anger that you felt at your mother for her demands. Now, you were partly justified in being angry at him because he was inefficient, but you also enjoyed seeing your mother approve of your tactics.

PATIENT: Yes, I did.

THERAPIST: The question is, why did you have to take all this round about way of dealing with both your parents? Why couldn't you be angry at your mother for her demands and equally angry at your father for his abortive intervention?

PATIENT:. . . I was always afraid of violence.

THERAPIST: Violence? Who's talking about violence?

PATIENT: Whenever people argue, whether it's my parents or others, I always think of violence—physical violence—and that's why I try to cover up my feelings.

THERAPIST: Physical violence?

PATIENT: Yes. I was always terrified of physical violence. I never had a fight with another kid, although many times I had fantasies that I would beat up anyone I wanted, yet I never did. I was a good athlete, but I avoided contact sports like football. I was a good swimmer.

THERAPIST: But why were you afraid?

PATIENT (*irritated*): I was afraid I'd get hurt.

THERAPIST: Since you never fought, how did you know you'd get hurt?

PATIENT: Well, my father was much bigger than I was.

THERAPIST: Did your father ever beat you up?

PATIENT: No.

THERAPIST: Did he ever hurt you?

PATIENT: No.

THERAPIST: So all this was in your mind.

PATIENT (*very irritated*): Yes.

THERAPIST: Why are you annoyed with me?

PATIENT: What do you mean?

THERAPIST: Right now, why?

PATIENT: I don't understand.

THERAPIST: Stop avoiding your irritation at me.

PATIENT: I'm not angry at what you're saying but at the way you go about asking me questions—"Why are you annoyed?" "Did he ever hurt you?"

THERAPIST: Does it remind you of anything?

PATIENT: Well, it's like that argument I had with my father.

THERAPIST: Precisely, but let's not forget that you won that argument.

PATIENT: That's it. . . . I feel angry because I'm not winning this argument with you.

THERAPIST: So although I remind you of your father, I seem to be somewhat different.

PATIENT: You bet you are.

THERAPIST: But this is helpful. Can't you see that there is a golden opportunity for you to express your anger without getting hurt right here?

PATIENT (*hesitating*): Yes, I can see that it makes sense.

THERAPIST: What strikes me, however, is that your father was very mild. Where did this notion of being hurt come from?

PATIENT: Well, you see, my father was a very successful business-man when I worked for him during the summer, as I mentioned. I was amazed to see how good my father was at work. Everybody admired him and was scared of him. I told you that we had intellectual discussions and his logic was always superior.

THERAPIST: Except when he was jealous of you, and you told me that at such times you detected flaws in his logic, didn't you?

PATIENT: Yes, I did.

THERAPIST: It is at those times, then, that you have those fantasies about violence?

PATIENT: Yes, exactly.

THERAPIST: So it's *you* who wants to hurt your father when you detect that he is in a weakened position—when he's jealous and when his logic fails him.

PATIENT: I don't like your putting it that way.

THERAPIST: I know. You don't like it because it's the truth, a truth that you distorted. You became the victim and you were afraid of being hurt by your father when in reality it was *you* who wanted to hurt *him*.

PATIENT: . . . I suddenly remembered a fantasy that I had when I was a child. I remembered being terrified of being swallowed in quicksand.

THERAPIST: And?

PATIENT: Well, I had the vision that I'd lose my pants, and that my father would come and rescue me.

THERAPIST: So from being aggressive toward him you become the victim, and it is he who rescues you.

PATIENT: Yes. It struck me that what you said was true.

THERAPIST: And what does this episode bring to mind? Why are you caught with your pants down?

PATIENT: Well, I have always had the fear, when I have the premature ejaculations, that maybe I have homosexual tendencies.

THERAPIST: Now, let's examine all this. What would your being a homosexual do for you?

PATIENT: If I'm a homosexual, I would avoid all the sexual problems with my wife and, as we have seen, all those sexual feelings in reference to my mother.

THERAPIST: True. What else?

PATIENT: Else?

THERAPIST: Yes.

PATIENT: . . . I don't know.

THERAPIST: So you have your cake and eat it too.

PATIENT: I don't understand. What do you mean?

THERAPIST: Just that. Now, look here . . . if being a homosexual would get you out of your problems with your wife and your mother, wouldn't it also get you out of your problems with your father?

PATIENT: My father?

THERAPIST: Yes. When your father is weak and you and your mother win, there is no difficulty; but when your father is logical and successful, as he was at the factory, then your father is strong. It's at such a time that you want to compete with him. Then you try to hurt him and try to beat him. Isn't that so?

PATIENT: Yes.

THERAPIST: It is then that you twist things around and that you become afraid that he will hurt you.

PATIENT: I agree.

THERAPIST: And fantasies of violence come to mind?

PATIENT: Yes.

THERAPIST: Now, what would a "strong" father do to his son, if he knew that his son had sexual feelings for his wife?

PATIENT: He'd be mad. He could hurt me.

THERAPIST: Precisely. So at such a time you cover up your anger and you become the victim, despite your fantasies about physical violence.

PATIENT: Hm.

THERAPIST: Now, what would a "strong father" do to his son if he knew that his son had sexual feelings for his wife?

PATIENT: Oh, after. Always after!

THERAPIST: Of course! Because if you become *weak* you can cover up your aggression; furthermore, it's your father who rescues you, isn't it?

PATIENT: Yes.

THERAPIST: At such a time *you* become the victim. You lose your pants and you have the idea that you are a homosexual.

PATIENT: Hm.

THERAPIST: So being a homosexual provides you with a perfect alibi, doesn't it?

PATIENT: Alibi?

THERAPIST: Yes, alibi. "Look, Dad, I'm a victim. I'm weak. You saved me. Furthermore I have no sexual feelings for your wife. You see, I'm a homosexual with my pants down."

PATIENT: Oh (*smiles*), I see!

THERAPIST: Yes, a pseudohomosexual, who deceives his father, pretending that he has no sexual feelings for women. At the same time, he tries to avoid sexual feelings for women when they become dangerous and make too many demands on him. Can't you see how this helps you "have your cake and eat it too?"

PATIENT: Oh, I see. (*looking very pleased with himself*)

THERAPIST: You look pleased with yourself!

PATIENT: Well, yes. I can understand things so much better. All this is very helpful. Actually, I have noticed many changes recently.

THERAPIST: Changes. In what way do you mean?

PATIENT: During the last two weeks I had good sex with Bonnie. Not only did I not have a premature ejaculation, but on the contrary we had good sex relations. Bonnie was happy. She had an orgasm. She was very pleased and so was I.

THERAPIST: I'm glad to hear about this. So maybe what we're doing here is helping you?

PATIENT: Oh, yes, indeed. Actually I was wondering how much longer I need to come here.

THERAPIST: It's a good question. How long do you think you need to come before we stop?

PATIENT: Well, not right away! Maybe we need two or three more sessions to tie up all the loose ends.

THERAPIST: I agree.

The session went on for a while longer. It was decided that they should meet three more times and then stop.

This interview speaks for itself. It is typical of the beginning of the end of STAPP. Not only are the transference feelings brought into the open, but also there is important problem-solving work being done in reference to the patient's pseudohomosexuality. Finally, the patient gives tangible evidence that his problem is being resolved when he refers to the improved relationship with his wife, and it is *he* who initiated the talk about termination. More about this subject, however, will be discussed in the following chapter.

CHAPTER 11

The Terminal Phase

EVIDENCE OF CHANGE AND DEVELOPMENT OF INSIGHT

It has been stated generally that termination of psychotherapy gives rise to feelings of loss, grief, and even guilt and anger, and that the way in which the therapist handles these feelings will determine the patient's ability to function independently after its ending. Such observations may be true in patients who face the termination of their analysis or long-term dynamic psychotherapy as well as in those patients receiving time-limited psychotherapy where the central issues, according to Mann (1973), involve loss and separations.

In STAPP, however, and particularly in those patients whose focus was an unresolved Oedipal issue, we have not witnessed the emergence of these powerful feelings or the struggles over the loss of their therapist. If anything, what is striking in STAPP patients is a prevailing pride in their accomplishments, and although the therapist is viewed in very positive terms and the ending of their relationship is faced with a certain degree of sadness, their ability to internalize their achievements as well as their therapists makes their separation a much easier task. More about this will be discussed in a later chapter.

As mentioned in the previous chapter, evidence of problem solving as well as differences in attitudes, behavioral patterns, and overall change in the patient are what the therapist should be looking for, and once he is convinced that they are taking place, this should signal to him that the treatment must soon come to an end.

What, then, should constitute evidence of change? What should the therapist be looking for in order to be convinced that it is actually taking place? First and foremost should be proof that the patient's attitude about his basic psychological problem, and its underlying Oedipal focus on which the therapy has been centered up to this point, has been altered. One of the ways in which the therapist can test whether this is the case is by asking the patient to explain his understanding of his own psychodynamics. In STAPP it is vital that by the end of the treatment both the therapist and the patient be clearly aware of the psychodynamics underlying the psychological difficulties. In addition, the therapist should ask the patient to give him specific examples of situations in which new attitudes and behavior patterns have been changed, and differences between the current and former ways in which the patient is dealing with key people in his environment. Finally, information should be obtained about the development of new relations, as well as the appearance of novel ways of handling old problems. The diminution or disappearance of past neurotic patterns should constitute tangible evidence that basic changes have indeed taken place and that some insight has been developed.

One of the best ways for the therapist to make these observations is to scrutinize the transference relationship. The demonstration of progressive independence, self-assurance, improved self-esteem, and less reliance on the therapist are important steps in the right direction. Here is an example:

A 26-year-old woman who complained of agoraphobia and hyperventilation had reacted somewhat regressively to her therapist's two-week absence in the early part of the therapy. She complained of an exacerbation in her symptoms, became tearful, and tended to act somewhat passive and dependent. During the subsequent interviews, however, considerable insight was obtained about her sensitivity to separations. It was clearly associated with her sailor father's frequent absences for naval tours of duty when she was young. She indicated that during these times she tended to push out of her mind her father's prospective separation and was shocked to find out that he was again planning to leave her. Much work had been done in the ensuing weeks discussing with her the importance of anticipatory mechanisms and emphasizing the maladaptive and destructive effects of her denials. When the therapist planned another separation from the patient after the tenth interview, her reaction to his absence was very different. She went on as follows:

PATIENT: Although I still don't like the idea of your going away, there is a part of me that is looking forward to it. I want to test my own reactions to see how I think and behave while you're not here. It would be a good preparation for the time when I won't be coming to see you any more.

THERAPIST: But we know that you were unhappy the last time that I was away.

PATIENT: Oh, yes. . . . I'm not proud of what happened the last time you went away. I behaved like a child. I used my symptoms to feel sorry for myself in the hope that you were going to change your plans. Now that was childish!

THERAPIST: You are too harsh on yourself. We know that you were sensitive to separation. There was, however, an element of manipulation, wasn't there?

PATIENT: Oh, yes. I know I'm manipulative and I also don't like this trait in me.

THERAPIST: I'm glad to hear it, and actually, it didn't work with me, did it?

PATIENT: No, I know. But I feel very different this time.

THERAPIST: Why is this so?

PATIENT: I think a great deal had to do with that hour when we talked about my father's frequent tours of duty, and when I told you about all the fuss I created that time when I was six years old. I remember clearly that my temper tantrum was aimed at making my dad feel sorry for me, and at that time it was successful because he postponed his trip for two whole days! In your case, on the other hand, my temper tantrum and my manipulation didn't work. You went away. At that time, I was furious because you didn't behave the way I wanted, but of course I soon realized how neurotic I was and how self-destructive all this behavior of mine was. (*It appears from this statement that a "true corrective emotional experience" had taken place.*) . . . I feel confident that this time I'll manage very well by myself.

THERAPIST: I have no doubt that you will.

Indeed she did.

Another aspect to which the therapist should pay attention has to do with the subtle changes in the patient's attitudes about his symptoms. Patients at such times refer to "not being as bothered" by their symptoms as in the past, or state that the symptoms did not have as much "impact" on them as they did previously. Since the symptoms do represent compromises or partial solutions of underlying conflicts, an improvement should signal that these very conflicts have been solved. A word of caution, however, should be said about the expectation that the symptoms should disappear completely before the therapy ends. This takes much time because patients tend to become accustomed to their symptoms, which turn into habits, easy to get used to and hard to give up completely.

Another area in which the therapist can observe changes taking place has to do with interpersonal relations. Not only should one pay attention to various alterations of preexisting patterns of behavior in old relations, but also any new relationship should always be scrutinized very carefully. Here is an example:

A 27-year-old female lab technician had sought psychotherapy because of a repetitive neurotic pattern in her relations with men which seemed to make her very anxious. Whenever she met a man, she would become very flirtatious and seductive. She would also pursue with unusual vigor any man who was reluctant to get involved with her. She always gave every indication that she was interested in having sexual relations, but as soon as he showed interest in her and asked her to have intercourse with him, she would act as if she had been insulted, she would become cold and sarcastic, and soon thereafter she would end the relationship. Several of her male friends became angry at this behavior of hers, and on occasion told her in no uncertain terms what they thought of her neurotic difficulties.

During STAPP, the same neurotic pattern was transferred onto her male therapist, who pointed out early during the treatment that her efforts to seduce him were thin disguises of repeating the pattern she had developed with men, and of finding an excuse to end her therapy. Her initial response to this kind of confrontation was anger, but she seemed to be intrigued by someone she could not manipulate. She did not run away.

As the therapy went on, the patterns of her neurotic behavior became progressively clear. The men to whom she was attracted were substitutes for her father. They all had the same physical build. Her rejection of them was an attempt to pacify her mother's expected rage, which she feared greatly. As she gained insight into her problems, she seemed to become progressively more relaxed, and her transference to her therapist became more positive.

During the ninth interview she casually mentioned meeting a new man at a cocktail party, but did not elaborate. The therapist, however, was very much interested in the appearance of a new social contact:

THERAPIST: Can you tell me something more about your new acquaintance?

PATIENT: There isn't very much to say. Bill is a nice fellow.

THERAPIST: This is interesting. This is the first time that you have referred to one of your male acquaintances by name. In the past you've always referred to them as "my friend," "my boyfriend," or "my man." I always had to ask you for their names and usually you seemed hesitant to give them to me. You preferred to keep them anonymous.

PATIENT: Yes, that's true. It's possible that there's something different about the way I feel for Bill.

THERAPIST: Shall we hear more about this, then?

PATIENT: Well, I noticed him during a cocktail party and I thought that he was attractive, but I did not go rushing over to him as I usually do.

THERAPIST: So this was different from the way we know you go about approaching men. Isn't it?

PATIENT: Possibly. I don't know. You see, Bill doesn't look like anyone else I know. I'm usually attracted to tall, blond men. Bill has a very handsome face, but he's somewhat short. He's no taller than I am, five feet nine or so, and he's on the stocky side. It was he who pursued me. He came over and started to talk to me. He invited me to have dinner with him. I accepted. I was flabbergasted.

THERAPIST: So, this is a new way of relating to a man?

PATIENT: Maybe. Recently I've been thinking a lot about my attraction to tall, blond men. I thought, "How childish!" Because Dad was tall and blond, there I go acting like a teenager; and you know, many a time I ended by going out with some dumb tall, blond man.

It was clear from this cautious description of her new relationship that her understanding of the dynamics of her Oedipal struggle was producing some tangible evidence that her relations were changing for the better.

As things developed, her relationship with Bill turned out to be meaningful and long-lasting, and it signaled the beginning of the end of her neurotic behavior patterns.

WHO INITIATES TERMINATION?

Whenever one deals with the issue of termination, one of course is confronted with the patient's proverbial ambivalent feelings about the loss of the therapist. As mentioned before, Mann (1973) is so impressed by termination that he structures his whole 12-session time-limited psychotherapy in preparation for its ending.

In contrast, we have no difficulty in terminating STAPP, which focuses on Oedipal issues. Although loss does play a role during the Oedipal period, it is not the devastating loss that occurs in patients who were fixated in earlier pregenital stages. Termination of their therapy is viewed by the majority of STAPP patients as the logical conclusion of this hard, problem-solving work.

Who, then, initiates discussion about terminating treatment? It is obvious that the decision to bring STAPP to an end should be primarily the therapist's, because he is more objective and in a better position to observe any changes taking place. In reviewing our cases, however, I was struck by the fact that in half of them it was the patient who first mentioned the possibility of ending. Here is an example:

A 26-year-old female graduate student, who had sought therapy because of anxiety attacks, commented on her therapist's prospective three-week European trip as follows:

PATIENT: I feel so different this time about your trip than I did about the last time you were gone. I've prepared myself for it. I've been anticipating it now for the last five weeks. When I first think of it

I feel a little unhappy, but then I start thinking about trying to do the work by myself. I say to myself, "After all, Margie, you'll be on your own when the therapy is over. Isn't this going to be a golden opportunity to see how well you can do by yourself without your therapist?" Actually, I remember an episode when I was seven, when my father and mother also went on a trip to Europe. At that time I threw a temper tantrum, begging them not to go. I remember that my mother was upset, but my father said that it would be good for me to be on my own. Actually, he was right. After they left I managed very well. During that time I also met Mary, who became my best friend; in addition, I became interested in my schoolwork and I got very good grades. Well, your going away brought all these things to mind. I plan to work hard on my thesis the next three weeks. I have a lot to do and I feel confident that I'll accomplish a lot.

THERAPIST: And how are your anxiety attacks? I haven't heard very much about them lately.

PATIENT: Well, I still feel anxious at times, but somehow I'm not bothered by this as much. I have the feeling that if all goes well while you're gone, it will be a sign that I'm ready to terminate my therapy. What do you think?

THERAPIST: I'm inclined to agree with you. It seems that most of the work which we set out to do has been done. Now you should put your self-understanding to work. From what you say, you seem to be ready to do it.

PATIENT: Yes, I am.

THERAPIST: So, shall we plan to have two more sessions after I return?

PATIENT: Okay, except if I have some problem come up while you're away which I can't deal with by myself.

THERAPIST: I understand, but do you think that there could be a problem which you would not be able to cope with by yourself?

PATIENT: To be honest with you, I don't think so. It is just that I am a bit hesitant. It's difficult to get used to this new freedom which I have discovered lately.

THERAPIST: I understand and I'm completely in agreement with you.

This example is fairly typical of the STAPP patient's initiating talk about termination of treatment. At first, it appears that thoughts about ending are somewhat vague, but as the patients start thinking about them, these thoughts become progressively more clear-cut and finally crystallize into the concrete decisions that they are ready to finish their therapy.

Of course, the therapist should be cautious about terminating the treatment of a patient who is fleeing so as to avoid facing his conflicts. This is a very rare phenomenon, but because it can take place at times, one should be on the alert and try to avoid it. The best guide to the therapist, therefore, should be his appraisal of the resolution of the patient's basic Oedipal problem. If he feels confident that this task has been accomplished, then the treatment should come to an end.

One of the common pitfalls into which many an inexperienced therapist tends to fall has to do with a lack of confidence about the speed of his own therapeutic achievement—"How could so much be accomplished in such a short time interval?" It is contrary to all the teachings about the long time that it takes for changes to take place. This unfortunate suspicion and false impression are responsible, in my opinion, for the unnecessary prolongation of treatment.

Another unfortunate attitude held by the therapist faced with the prospect of termination has to do with his own omnipotence—"How can a patient function without the therapist's help?" The possibility that this may be true wounds some therapists' egos, and they try to find excuses to continue the therapy.

ABSENCE OF AMBIVALENCE ABOUT ENDING TREATMENT

Some STAPP patients do not initiate the talk about termination, being somewhat more passive, or enjoying the treatment so much that they leave its ending in the hands of their therapists. In that case it is the therapist's task to broach this subject. Here is an example:

A 24-year-old male accountant started his eleventh interview as follows:

PATIENT: I had a very good week. The last session here was most interesting. Everything seemed to fall into place. I had never before realized how much I had set up these triangular situations, always being interested in unavailable women, always flirting with the girls of my best friends. Last time, this episode with Wanda was the clincher. (*He was referring to a situation when he tried to seduce the fiancée of his best friend one week before she was to be married, and he was to be the best man.*) What made a lot of difference was your statement that there was "a whole world of *available* women to choose from." I thought about that during the week, and suddenly I felt free. "Yes," I said, "a whole world of available women and I go about compulsively getting myself entangled in these triangular interactions, always losing and always endangering my friendships." It was like being in a morass. It was this neurotic compulsion of mine which had so much to do with my mother and which I had been unable to shake for all this time. By the way, I had a date this last week.

THERAPIST: Oh, I see. Can we hear about it?

PATIENT: Well, yes. It was with this girl at the office whom I had known for quite some time, but I had not paid much attention to her because I knew that she wasn't going steady with anyone. She's a nice girl. Her name is Dora. She's not as beautiful as these other women I've been telling you about, but she's quite nice and very bright. Well, last Wednesday after I had been thinking about our session, I said to myself, "Why not take Dora out for dinner? She's a nice kid." I did, and you know what? We had a heck of a good time. The main thing about it was that I felt free. I didn't have to look over my shoulder to see if a boyfriend or a husband or whoever, you know, was suddenly going to come in and catch us. I felt good. I felt grown-up.

THERAPIST: Hm!

PATIENT: Another thing of interest was that I did not think of sex right away. I enjoyed talking with Dora. Not that I'm not sexually interested in her. No, far from it. She has a nice figure. But I didn't feel the need to rush into things. Dora is a real person, not exotic, not flamboyant, like all these other women, but solid and bright, a fine human being. I feel very good about her and about this newly found freedom.

THERAPIST: So when shall we stop?

PATIENT: Stop what?

THERAPIST: Stop psychotherapy.

PATIENT (*appalled, stupified*): Therapy? My God, no! Now that everything is going on so well?

THERAPIST: Precisely. This may be the best time indeed.

PATIENT: But why? There's so much more to talk about. I have so many other problems. I have my doubts that I'll be able to maintain this newly found freedom. My God! There I am telling you that I feel better and the next thing that happens is that you talk about ending this treatment. I don't want to end. I like it. It has done me a lot of good. I have a very different picture of myself. I have a clear understanding of the origin of my difficulties which is so true. I can see how I have displaced my feelings for my mother and my father onto every friend of mine and his girl. I don't need to do all this any longer. I've learned a great deal.

THERAPIST: Yes. It's because of all these things that I think that we shall stop soon. (*The patient went on complaining for another 10 minutes or so. He then burst out laughing*):

PATIENT: I know what I'm doing and it's silly. All this time I'm trying to convince you, not me, that I need more therapy. I do it, as I said before, because I like this treatment and because I respect you and all the help that you gave me. I know it's foolish to try to convince you about something that I know is wrong. I know that I have solved the problem you and I set up to work on. This example that I gave you about Dora is evidence that I have changed. I want to go on, but I know I must stop because there is very little more to be done here. It's time to stand on my own two feet and be my own boss.

This statement is fairly typical and quite moving. In a variety of ways STAPP patients recognize clearly when their problem has been solved. They may procrastinate for a while, but they soon realize that it is useless to prolong a situation which seems to be rapidly coming to an end. What is ironic may be that the need to prolong their therapy is due primarily to the positive transference feelings for their therapists and the strength of the therapeutic alliance, two of the cardinal aspects of the STAPP technique.

STAPP patients seem to work up to the last minutes of the last hour. They prefer to problem-solve, and although they do mention feeling sad because they will miss their therapist, they also stress their pleasure at having done the job well, and look forward to being on their own. There is none of the ambivalence and anger at the prospective separation which are encountered during the termination of psychoanalysis or long-term supportive psychotherapeutic intervention. The reasons for this ambivalence and anger are obvious—such patients have difficulties with pregenital characterological issues. STAPP patients, as we know, do not; therefore, they do not experience any ambivalence at the prospect of termination. Their sadness is appropriate, and it is shared by their therapists as well.

PART THREE

RESULTS

CHAPTER 12

Instruction in STAPP

A few words should be spoken now about teaching STAPP methods. From what has been discussed already, it should be fairly obvious that this kind of brief therapy can easily be taught to relatively inexperienced therapists if certain preconditions are followed very rigorously.

CRITERIA FOR BECOMING A STAPP THERAPIST

From my own observations of the supervision of 70 therapists representing such disciplines as psychiatry, psychology, social work, and nursing during the last 25 years, I can state categorically that the main difficulty in learning to use STAPP has had more to do with certain misconceptions about the superiority of long-term psychotherapy which were rigidly embedded in the minds of our trainees, and which they were reluctant to give up, than with anything else, including their relative inexperience. This problem was resolved when we decided to make instruction in STAPP an elective part of our training program and offer it to our trainees early so as to avoid their being thoroughly indoctrinated in dogmatic points of view and in preconceived and narrow-minded ideas which tended to obscure their ability to make meaningful observations which interfered with their learning.

It is of interest, therefore, to note that these therapists shared with their STAPP patients a common characteristic: they were *mo-*

tivated to change. This crucial criterion for patient selection turned
out to be the most valuable asset of the therapists. Their enthusiasm
proved to be the most important ingredient for the successful treatment of their STAPP patients, because it enabled them to create a
therapeutic alliance which, despite all the resistances and difficulties encountered, withstood all stresses and strains and contributed
greatly to the ultimate success of their treatment.

A question which is usually asked has to do with the specific
requirements necessary for someone to become a STAPP therapist.
Generally speaking, in addition to good motivation and possession
of an open mind, it is important that STAPP therapists be familiar
with psychodynamic theory and, of course, be well acquainted with
the technical requirements of this kind of treatment. Beyond that,
however, instruction in STAPP should involve intensive individual
or group supervision of the therapeutic interaction with a suitable
patient.

THE NATURE OF STAPP SUPERVISION

In my chapter entitled "Learning and Teaching STAPP" that
will appear in the *Proceedings of the First and Second International
Symposia for Short-Term Dynamic Psychotherapy* (Davanloo, in
press), I discussed in some detail the special educational aspects involved in STAPP supervision. Here I would like to summarize
briefly what was included in that discussion and to add certain innovations which we initiated more recently.

First, the supervisor selects an appropriate candidate and interviews him, preferably on videotape, to be sure that he or she fulfills
the criteria for selection and has an identifiable Oedipal focus.
Then, he meets with the supervisee and discusses with him any
specific difficulties which are likely to be encountered. Finally, the
supervisor enumerates the various technical aspects of STAPP and
outlines the specific criteria for a successful outcome.

From then on each interview is discussed in detail, with constant attention paid to the collection of pertinent material, to the
utilization of the transference, and to a concentration on the therapeutic focus. The use of anxiety-provoking confrontations and interpretations is discussed and the careful avoidance of the pregenital characterological issues is emphasized.

The student is told to collect his data carefully, particularly during the early part of the therapy, to enable him to use specific details obtained from the patient when he makes his interpretations later on during the treatment.

The supervisee is encouraged to take written notes and to pay special attention to any shifts occurring in the patient's recounting of his past life experiences, or to sudden shifts in the transference relationship as a result of defensive maneuvers. Countertransference feelings also need to be scrutinized, particularly when the therapist concentrates on clarifying the Oedipal focus, which may in time be colored by his own feelings and may stir up some trouble if not handled correctly. During such times, the supervisor should be very careful to support the therapist in such a way as to help him distinguish clearly between his own countertransference feelings and the patient's neurotic interactions. He must be careful, however, not to turn the supervisory sessions into psychotherapy for the trainee. If indeed this becomes necessary—and in my experience it has occurred only once—the trainee's difficulties should be openly discussed with him, and he should be encouraged to seek psychiatric help for himself.

Other areas of difficulty which are likely to be encountered in supervising STAPP therapists include their reluctance to deal with transference feelings as early as possible, and their tendency to be unwilling to initiate the talk of termination even when all evidence points to a resolution of the patient's problem. I think this latter difficulty has to do with doubts on the part of a supervisee of his own therapeutic capabilities, as well as his liking of the patient and his reluctance to separate from him.

The rapid production of rich material by the patient during the early phase of STAPP may create at times difficulties for the student therapist. Having been thoroughly indoctrinated as to what should and should not be done by his supervisors of long-term psychotherapy, many students develop certain preconceived ideas which at times are difficult to change. What I am referring to here is what the therapist thinks ought to be taking place under his very eyes. Thus it is important to emphasize to the students that STAPP has been developed as a result of a systematic observation of what is taking place in the patient, and not from some theoretical generalization about psychopathology.

If the student therapist is able to follow objectively what his patient is presenting to him and to utilize the techniques which I have already described, he will discover for himself that this kind of therapy is not as difficult to learn as he might have expected.

Recently, one of our trainees described her experience as follows: "I was amazed to see so much fantasy material flowing out of the patient. He reminded me of a horse galloping along. At first I had a tendency to try to restrain him; the result was that his gallop became uneven or jerky, but it continued nevertheless. When finally it occurred to me that I should let him carry on at his own pace, everything went smoothly from then on. The gallop slowly turned into a trot and finally came to a complete stop. I was sure, at this point, that we had reached the time for a transference clarification. As soon as I did it, I was surprised to see him start trotting along and soon galloping at high speed all over again. It was really marvelous. It was a great experience." And then she added, "You see, I always liked horseback riding!" I was sure that she was as good at riding as she was at treating patients.

THE USE OF VIDEOTAPE

I have always been very enthusiastic about the use of videotapes, which I have called the "microscope of the psychiatrist" because they have enabled our specialty during the last few years to become a truly scientific discipline (Sifneos, 1975a).

Videotapes are used to evaluate patients, to study the outcome of short-term dynamic therapies, and to demonstrate the treatment process and the technical requirements of these therapeutic modalities. In addition, they proved to be an invaluable asset in the education of our students.

We used videotapes to record the treatment of several STAPP patients, presenting and discussing them systematically with our trainees. The ability to make short-term predictions of what would take place during the following session was emphasized. After a thorough discussion of various happenings during the interview, the students speculated about what reactions the patient might manifest in the next session. This kind of teaching exercise proved to be one of the most popular with our residents. Furthermore, videotape demonstrations to our students of STAPP patients in follow-up interviews, some several years after their treatment had been terminated, were the best scientific documentation of the value of this kind of therapy.

It was up to the students to decide for themselves whether or not the treatment had been successful and to make comparisons between the patient's patterns of behavior at the time of the initial evaluation and long after the therapy had terminated.

One of the innovations which I introduced recently in the teaching of our trainees involves the use of videotapes during the supervisory sessions. The resident who is willing to cooperate agrees to treat a STAPP patient on videotape. A suitable patient from our research pool is then selected who also agrees to be videotaped, to sign an informed consent form, and to be interviewed by two independent evaluators so as to set up a baseline of his or her behavior patterns. This is utilized in pre- and posttreatment comparisons.

During the supervisory session the resident usually presents a summary of his interview with the patient, emphasizing the areas in which he has certain technical questions. He then selects certain parts of the videotape which demonstrate his technique. Since the supervisory session is also videotaped, we have an opportunity to have on record all the interactions that take place between the patient and his therapist, as well as between the therapist and the supervisor. Furthermore, after the supervisory session is over, the therapist has the opportunity to review both his own interview and the comments of his supervisor during the teaching session. Here is an example:

During the psychotherapy of a female STAPP patient with a very gifted first-year resident, it became clear that the patient was experiencing progressively sexualized transference feelings for her therapist. She became more and more seductive and in many ways tried to demonstrate how attracted she felt to our trainee. Although he was somewhat reluctant and felt a little embarrassed by all this behavior, keeping in mind that he had no experience in dealing explicitly with transference feelings, the resident decided nevertheless, as a result of my urging, that it was time to help the patient clarify her own transference feelings. He chose, however, to emphasize the nature of her feelings for her mother, which he felt were similar to those she experienced for him, because during the early part of the treatment she had used the same words to describe both her mother and himself. It was clear that he missed the point, to both the patient's and his supervisor's consternation. When this part of the videotape was played back, it became quite clear to the resident what had happened. He could see the patient's disappointment at his transference confrontation. When we discussed his countertransference feelings, he readily admitted that he had felt embarrassed by the patient's seductiveness, for which he was prepared intellectually, but could not bring himself to deal with appropriately because of his own feelings for her. The videotaped supervisory session brought his dilemma clearly into focus. He was prepared, therefore, to deal with the transference explicity during the following sessions.

The patient appeared subdued during the early part of the next interview. She looked sad and disappointed, and her general behavior was much less seductive than it had been during the previous hour. After a while, however, she again alluded to her feelings about the therapist. At this point the resident decided to intervene. He was able to draw very expertly a parallel between her feelings for her father, for her boyfriend, for her boss at work, and for him. The impact of this skillful interpretation was immediate. On the screen one could see the patient brighten up and admit her deep disappointment at his clarifications the previous week. From then on the psychotherapy proceeded eventfully and ended successfully. A six-month follow-up, also recorded on videotape, showed that the patient had improved dramatically, that she was able to utilize what she had learned during her therapy, and that she had a clear understanding of her relations to her parents as well as to key men and women in her daily life. All in all, the criteria listed for a successful therapeutic outcome had clearly been met. One cannot overemphasize the value of videotaping supervision, of videotaping STAPP, or, as far as it goes, of videotaping any other kind of psychotherapy. All in all, it can be stated categorically that STAPP is one of the best kinds of treatment to use for teaching psychotherapy to our trainees. Because of its specific technical requirements and its shortness of duration, it offers enormous advantages not only for educational and therapeutic purposes but also for research.

Another advantage of videotape is its use in continuous psychiatric education courses. We have used a variety of tapes to illustrate the evaluation of STAPP patients as well as the technical requirements and outcomes of STAPP treatment in several of our workshops. The comments of various participants representing all the mental health professions have been invaluable not only in improving our educational program but also in improving STAPP itself.

I am indebted to Dr. Louis Bloomingdale, who has attended two of our workshops, for graciously permitting me to include his comments here. This is what he had to say about STAPP after viewing several of our videotaped interviews:

Analysis of STAPP Technique

1. Focus on specific *problem*.

   This is a taboo in psychoanalysis as leading to intellectualization. It provides the patient with a more familiar mode of usual learning and divests the transference of some magical, pre-Oedipal factors induced by the "mysteriousness" in usual psychoanalytic psychotherapy.

2. "This is very interesting." "This is intriguing."

   These statements by the therapist show his interest (taboo in psychoanalysis); the patient's curiosity is aroused, collaboration is encouraged, and the groundwork for intersession and postsession "working through" is stimulated.

3. "What do *you* think?" "What are *you* telling me?" "Don't run away from *your* problem." "It's not my job to answer *your* questions."

   Instead of making interpretations and usually discounting the patient's own interpretations as "not true associations," the patient's independence is fostered and, again, the patient feels able to "work through" by himself. This enhances the patient's responsibility and reduces the authoritarianism of the therapist, encouraging less regression.

4. Note taking of specific material.
   a. This reinforces "learning" and "problem-solving" concepts.

   b. The patient is taken seriously.
   c. The Oedipal material and specific emergence of "pre-
      conscious nodal points" are emphasized by notes being
      taken, which are later used in recapitulation.

5. Support is provided by the therapist for the emergence of
   preconscious material.

   The therapist indicates his empathy with the embarrassment and stresses that the "work" is difficult but very
   worthwhile.

6. The therapist asks, "Why do you think . . . ?"

   Psychotherapists are instructed not to ask "why?"
   since, obviously, the patient doesn't know why. In STAPP,
   it is communicated that the patient can answer "why?" by
   permitting memories to emerge from the preconscious. In
   "working through," the patient has learned to pose and answer his own question "why?" which patients in usual
   psychotherapy have been taught not to ask (although they
   may use the same technique if psychotherapy has been effective).

7. Regression is discouraged, as is discussion of pre-Oedipal
   characterological problems.

   While in psychoanalysis regression is encouraged as
   "being in the service of the ego," it often is not useful.
   With these patients, in STAPP the discussion of pre-
   Oedipal material is a defense against Oedipal anxiety.

8. The therapist forces the patient to accept responsibility for
   feelings and fantasies.

   This integrates the "internal self" so it grows as the influence of internalized objects is decreased. These introjects
   are replaced somewhat by the incorporation of the therapist
   as a "problem-solving helper," so that there is not the intense feeling of loss ordinarily experienced by the ex-
   ternalization of introjects.

9. Recapitulation.

   By the therapist's providing a cognitive summary, the
   patient is encouraged to embrace the concept that a problem can be solved with a tangible "solution."

10. The therapist labels all "parent-transference links" as soon as they are identified.

    This prevents regression in the transference to pre-Oedipal levels.

11. The therapist continuously applies pressure relating to the infantile triangle.

12. This is what really seems to be meant by the term "anxiety-provoking." It results in a special focusing of attention on a nodal point of balance forcing preconscious emergence of a repressed idea (with anxiety often manifested by alternating lateral hand and/or forearm movements, which I have rarely seen in usual psychotherapy, where anxiety is usually expressed in gross movements of the total body or extremities, or changes in tonal vocal quality). These alternating hand movements seem to express vacillation between "instinctual drive" on the one side versus "defense" (repression) on the other. In these carefully selected patients who have good ego strength, the anxiety is resolved *by the patient* in the breakthrough and by the therapist-supported acceptance of repressed ideas.

In addition to these observations, Dr. Bloomingdale made a detailed study of the patient's movements during several interviews. It appears that hand and arm movements seem to be correlated consistently with the material which is brought up by the patient. It is evident from all this that nonverbal communication plays a significant role in STAPP, and more attention will be paid to its study in the future.

One cannot end a discussion of the use of videotapes in STAPP without mentioning their importance in the research about the outcome of the therapy. It should be obvious that the opportunity which independent evaluators can have in observing the patient at the time of their evaluations, in viewing the interviews during the whole course of the therapy, and, above all, in scrutinizing the changes which have taken place after the treatment has come to an end is valuable. The test of a successful outcome of any psychotherapy should lie in its ability to demonstrate to objective observers the results which have been observed in long-term follow-up interviews.

I suspect that the resistance which has been encountered in the use of videotapes, particularly in the past, has to do with the insecurity of the therapists whose techniques, and results are being scrutinized by independent evaluators.

Recently I used the technique in follow-up interviews by showing the patients a tape of one of their earlier STAPP interviews. On the upper quadrant of the video screen the old interview is shown while in the rest of the screen one can observe the patient's reactions to is. Usually the patient can stop the tape and comment about it.

It is very impressive to witness the reactions of the patients under those circumstances. Some appear to be annoyed at their past performance, others are amused, and some are irritated to view their neurotic behavior. Few remember their emotions exactly, while some have completely forgotten about what had happened during a specific session or their emotions in reference to various aspects of their treatment.

One patient, while looking at herself struggling to deal with a difficult conflict in reference to her mother, cheered when she viewed herself dealing with her in an appropriate way. Another patient who observed his gesticulating exclaimed that he was "a true representative of his country of origin."

CHAPTER 13

The Outcome of
STAPP

Psychotherapeutic outcome can be seen as having three distinct dimensions, as proposed by Strupp and Hadley (1977) in their attempt to set up a conceptual model to evaluate mental health. These should be kept clearly in mind whenever one attempts to assess the results of psychotherapy. They involve society, the patient, and the therapist. Society tends to view mental health in terms of observed behavior and social conformity. The patient, on the other hand, considers his own well-being first and foremost and equates his own mental health with it. Finally, the therapist tends to view the patient's functioning according to his own theoretical model of personality structure.

In considering the outcome of patients who have received STAPP according to this model, it can be seen that most of these patients demonstrated observable behavior which was clearly accepted by society, and that they felt much better about themselves. Thus there seemed to be improvement from both the social and idiosyncratic points of view. Finally, since these patients were chosen because they were considered by their evaluators to be structurally sound and because they had improved in the opinions of their therapists and the independent observers of follow-up, it was clear that as a result of STAPP the majority had attained a high level of mental health functioning according to the Strupp and Hadley criteria, not only by the end of their treatment but continuing many years subsequent to its termination.

Malan (1976c), in his discussion of the validation of brief dynamic psychotherapy, was able to confirm better than anyone else in the field the value of this kind of treatment by assessing its outcome in terms of dynamic changes occurring at the time of follow-up, matched with criteria for improvement specified at the time of the patient's evaluation by uncontaminated judges. This type of research should be done not only by other investigators interested in the field of brief dynamic psychotherapy but also by those who believe in, but who have not demonstrated adequately, the value of long-term dynamic psychotherapy.

EARLY STUDIES

In 1960 and again in 1964, I presented the findings of follow-up interviews with patients who were treated with STAPP (Sifneos, 1961, 1965). The results can be summarized as follows: The patients reported that (1) they had achieved a moderate symtomatic relief, (2) psychotherapy was a "new learning experience," (3) their self-esteem had improved strikingly, (4) they had overcome the crisis which was instrumental in bringing them to the clinic, and (5) their expectations of the therapeutic outcome had become more realistic. Furthermore, it appeared that, although they had experienced positive feelings for their therapists, the patients attributed the success of their treatment primarily to their own efforts. Generally speaking, they felt no need for further psychotherapy. At that time, although we were quite encouraged by these findings, we thought that STAPP provided only limited intrapsychic changes. We did, however, decided to investigate the therapeutic outcome more systematically by setting up a controlled study of patients chosen according to our selection criteria and treated according to the technical requirements that are by now very familiar to the reader.

The patients were seen by two independent evaluators before and after their therapy. They were designated as either "experimental" or "control" and were matched according to age and sex. The control patients waited for the approximate period of time that it took for their experimental counterparts to be treated and were then seen again in order to assess any changes which had taken place while they were waiting. Following this, they were also offered STAPP. After the termination of their treatment, the results obtained with them were compared with those obtained from the experimental patient group who had been treated without having to wait. Both groups were followed as long as possible.

In 1968 the results of this controlled study were presented at the Ciba Symposium on the Role of Learning in Psychotherapy and appear in the volume by the same title (Sifneos, 1968a). In summary, 35 experimental and 36 control patients were studied, but 2 control patients were lost at the end of their working period. Unfortunately, many of the patients were students who left the Boston area after they finished therapy and were lost for follow-up study. Nevertheless, 14 experimental and 18 control patients were seen after the end of their treatment. The majority in both groups showed "moderate" or "complete" resolution of the emotional conflicts that were responsible for their difficulties. In addition, there was evidence of improved self-esteem in 30 out of the total of 32 patients, of self-understanding in 27 out of the 32, and of new learning and problem solving in 24 out of the 32. Finally, 23 of the 32 patients had a moderate symptomatic improvement.

It is of interest to note that after the end of their waiting period, the control patients showed no evidence that any change had taken place, except that several showed some symptomatic improvement as a result of some accidental event that occured while they were waiting. Despite this improvement, these patients did not lose their motivation for change since they realized only too well that their symptomatic improvement was accidental and that they had developed no insight whatsoever as to the real causes of their difficulties.

Long-term follow-up of up to 4 years for 21 patients showed the following results:

Moderate symptomatic relief	58%
Improved self-esteem	82%
New learning	77%
Improved interpersonal relations	77%
Improved problem-solving capacity	72%

Increased self-understanding   91%
Development of new attitudes and behavior patterns   86%

Although the numbers are small, these findings were impressive and encouraged us to pursue our investigation of the results of STAPP.

PSYCHOTHERAPEUTIC OUTCOME

One of the steps which were taken had to do with the specification of criteria for symptomatic improvement. These were considered under three main categories of change: (1) intrapsychic, (2) interpersonal, and (3) psychodynamic.

In my book *Short-Term Psychotherapy and Emotional Crisis* (Sifneos, 1972) I discussed in some detail these three categories of criteria for psychotherapeutic outcome.

The advantages of utilizing specific outcome criteria for psychotherapy research cannot be overemphasized. For example, we used outcome criteria not only to study the results of STAPP in the psychiatric clinic of the Beth Israel Hospital in Boston but also to investigate the outcome of other kinds of psychotherapies (Leeman, 1975). Having excluded those patients who were receiving STAPP and were being studied systematically, I decided to compare two homogeneous groups of patients, one receiving long-term psychotherapy of one or two years' duration and the second receiving a kind of brief psychotherapy which, although not similar to STAPP as far as technical requirements were concerned, was nevertheless more focused than long-term treatment. We refer to this kind of brief treatment as "brief psychotherapy (other types)." The study observed 18 patients received this type of brief therapy and 35 being treated with long-term psychotherapy by 14 different therapists.

The results of these investigations pointed to the discovery that symptomatic improvement occurred in more than half of both groups (68% of the long-term and 61% of the short-term patients), but motivation, self-esteem, and interpersonal relations seemed to improve more in the brief psychotherapy patients than in those receiving long-term treatment. Although it is possible that these changes tend not to reflect differences between brief and long-term therapy but rather identify patients who improve early irrespective of the therapy they receive, they are nevertheless significant.

Our most recent systematic investigation of the outcome of STAPP patients will be reported briefly here. In summary, all patients from the psychiatric clinic of the Beth Israel Hospital who fulfilled the criteria for selection who were thought to have an unresolved Oedipal problem, and who agreed to work on it in order to resolve it were interviewed by two independent evaluators. Their findings were reported during our research conference and were discussed in detail. If all members of the research group agreed that the patients were good STAPP candidates, they were accepted for our research study. If there was disagreement between the two evaluators, the case was discussed by the research group. Occasionally, despite an agreement between the evaluators, if enough doubts were raised by the members of the research group, the patient was excluded from the project and was placed in a "special" category. He was treated with STAPP nevertheless.

As in our previous studies, the patients were designated as either "experimental" or "control." The experimental patients were treated immediately while the controls waited. After the end of their therapy, the experimental patients were seen by a new, "uncontaminated" evaluator and by one of the two original evaluators in an effort to assess the results of the treatment and to see whether or not the outcome criteria specified for that patient during his evaluation had been fulfilled.

The patients were seen in follow-up interviews whenever possible on a yearly basis by one and, at times, two evaluators. The control patients waited approximately two to five months (which is the approximate length of time of STAPP). They usually were selected from a group of patients seeking treatment in the clinic during the period January–June, when most of the therapists had no time readily available for treatment, having filled their therapy schedules during the July to January period.

Following the waiting period the control patients were seen again by the evaluators to ascertain what changes had taken place without benefit of treatment. After this evaluation they were assigned to their STAPP therapists, and after its termination they were seen in follow-up interviews similar to those of their experimental counterparts.

OUTCOME CRITERIA

Every effort was made by the follow-up evaluators to rate the patients according to nine outcome criteria, which will be described briefly, as well as to obtain tangible examples of change, to make sure that dynamic changes had taken place, and to determine whether the following outcome criteria had been fulfilled and the predisposing Oedipal conflicts resolved.

The outcome criteria were (1) symptoms both psychological and physical, (2) interpersonal relations with key people in the patient's environment, (3) self-esteem, (4) development of new attitudes, (5) new learning, (6) problem solving, (7) self-understanding, (8) work or academic performance. In addition, the most important criterion involved (9) observation about changes in the individual basic predisposing factors responsible for and underlying the patient's problems. This has been referred to as SIP (specific internal predisposition). The evaluators also obtained information about the patients' overall view of their STAPP as well as about their feelings for their therapists.

The scoring for the outcome criteria was done as follows: The first eight criteria, with 50% of the total score, were given 6–7 for "recovery," 4–5 for "much better," 2–3 for "little better," and −1, 0, or 1 for "unchanged or worse." The ninth SIP criterion received the second 50% of the total score.

Thus, for example, a patient who was rated as having 6 for changes in symptoms, 7 for interpersonal relations, 6 for self-esteem, 5 for new attitudes, 5 for new learning, 5 for problem solving, 6 for self-understanding, and 4 for work performance, for 44 points divided by the 8 criteria, received a 5.5 for the first 50% of the total. If he got a 6.5 for SIP for the second 50% of the total, the final score was 12 (5.5 + 6.5). Thus a patient's total score of 11–14 signified "recovery," 7–11 "much better," 3–7 "little better," and −1 to 2 "unchanged" or "worse."

RECENT STAPP STUDY

Out of a total of 50 patients who had unresolved Oedipal conflicts, 36 were designated as "experimental" and 14 as "control." Of this total, 42 were females and 8 males. Some of the patients in our recent study had both the "evaluations" and follow-up interviews videotaped as well as the whole process of their therapy.

Fourteen control patients were seen at the end of their waiting period. In 11 of these there were no changes discernible as far as the nine outcome criteria were concerned. Three patients were scored as having had some symtomatic improvement as a result of environmental changes and were thought to be a "little better."

Here is an example:

A 25-year-old graduate student came to the clinic referred by her roommate because of depression and anxiety as a result of her procrastination and, in particular, her inability to decide whether or not she should marry her boyfriend. Her roommate, having been an "experimental" patient who was treated successfully with STAPP, recommended the psychiatric clinic to the patient and emphasized that there was no waiting in receiving treatment.

The patient was also thought to be a good STAPP candidate, having fulfilled the selection criteria and having been assessed as showing an unresolved Oedipal conflict, but she was told that she might have to wait since the patients were assigned at random to the experimental or control groups. She was disappointed to learn about this because she was eager to start her therapy.

It turned out that indeed she was a "control" patient and had to wait for five months for her experimental counterpart to be treated. When she was seen at the end of her waiting period she mentioned that she was not depressed anymore, her anxiety had disappeared, and she felt well. We of course inquired as to the cause of this symptomatic improvement, which took place without the benefit of therapy. This is what she said:

PATIENT: After I was seen here and had finished with my interviews I was told by the secretary that I would probably have to wait for several months. I felt very, very angry, thinking that the clinic was discriminating at some patients like myself, while treating others without any waiting, so I took matters in my own hands. I returned to my dorm, having bought a bottle of Scotch. I got drunk. Then flipped a coin, saying, "Heads I marry my boy friend and tails I don't." Heads came, and I decided to get married. It was the right decision, my anxiety disappeared, and I am happy.

EVALUATOR: Well, what else can we do for you?

PATIENT: When do I start my therapy? Don't tell me that I have to wait some more time.

EVALUATOR: You mean you are still interested in being treated?
PATIENT: Of course I am. I still don't know why I had that problem.
Why I was procrastinating. I want to find out the answer. After
all, it was all luck, because it would have been a catastrophe if
tails had fallen.

It is clear that the patient's motivation to change and to understand herself was strong. Nothing basic and taken place for her except that her symptoms had disappeared. She really wanted to understand the reasons for her difficulties so as to make sure that they
would not recur at some future time.

After the control patients were treated with STAPP, eight had
scores putting them in the "recovered" category and two were "much
better." Four patients decided to withdraw after the end of their
waiting period because of various realistic reasons, but, unfortunately, they had to be considered "lost" as far as our study was
concerned.

Of the 36 experimental patients, 21 had "recovered," 9 were
"much better," 3 were "little better," and 3 were designated "unchanged" and their therapy was considered to have been a failure.

Thus, of the 46 patients who were treated with STAPP (both
experimental and control), 29, or 63%, had "recovered" while 11, or
23%, were "much better."

Although the numbers may be small, they are nevertheless significant.

There are numerous problems associated with the systematic investigation of outcome studies. Because of these complexities many
potential investigators have been so discouraged that they arrived at
the erroneous conclusion that research of this kind was not practical,
while others were so perfectionistic in their approach they they became bogged down in details, missing the proverbial forest for the
trees.

We are aware that numbers do not reveal the whole story and
that outcome criteria may not give the total picture of the changes
which have taken place; nevertheless, our research team discussed
at length the nature of our criteria and we developed a consensus
about their specific meaning, particularly in reference to the most
important SIP criterion.

Difficulties which we encountered included, as mentioned, the loss of four control patients who withdrew at the end of the waiting period. Since many of our patients were students who finished their studies and left the Boston area, this seems to be an unavoidable problem. Also, the ability to bring back patients for a long-term follow-up interview is an exceedingly difficult problem in the United States because of the size of the country and the distances which are involved. A similar study of short-term dynamic psychotherapy in Norway (Husby, 1985a, b, and c) was much more successful than ours in that respect.

Another problem had to do with the efforts of one follow-up evaluator interview on the second interview. Many of these difficulties have been discussed at length in our paper "Ongoing outcome research on short-term dynamic psychotherapy" (Sifneos et al., 1980).

Our failures have been scrutinized and have been most instructive. Despite our efforts to assess the patients' "motivation for change" as thoroughly as possible, in two of our experimental patients who were rated as being only a "little better" and two who were unchanged we failed to evaluate this selection criterion adequately.

One of them also terminated her treatment prematurely at the time her therapist left for his summer vacation. When seen in follow-up, she was rated as having been better. Three years later, however, it was thought that she was essentially unchanged. She continued to live close to her parents and seemed to be fairly isolated from other people, yet she seemed fairly content with her status quo.

The second patient also seemed to have made considerable progress when seen after the end of her therapy. At that time her symptoms had improved considerably, but, having reverted to her old ways of functioning, she was rated as unchanged by both evaluators who saw her four years later. In both of these patients it was thought that no clear-cut parent-transference connections had been attempted during the course of their treatment. This may have contributed to the lack of a clear-cut resolution of their Oedipal conflicts. It was obvious, however, that only a temporary and superficial symptomatic improvement took place, which could not be maintained for long.

Another patient was one who was offered STAPP but who steadfastly resisted dealing with her transference feelings, and who was able very adroitly to avoid talking about them despite her therapist's efforts. Although there was no change in her symptoms of mild depression, or any improvement in her relations with her husband, she was rated by two evaluators as having been a "little better" with regard to self-understanding, problem solving, and self-esteem. Thus it is possible that transference reistance may have been the main stumbling block in all three of these patients. The question remains, of course, whether these difficulties resulted from the inexperience of the therapists or from the fact that the patients were not appropriate candidates for this kind of therapy and should not have been selected to receive it. As the therapy progressed and their anxiety mounted, their motivation, particularly in reference to dealing with transference feelings, faltered, and the therapy produced only a small improvement.

Finally, a patient at the end of her therapy seemed to have improved and one year later reported improved ability to deal with her parents, "more able to stand up for my own opinions and recognize my emotions, and more objective about my relations with men." Subsequently, following her father's hospitalization for a manic episode, the patient also had a psychotic illness and was diagnosed as having a bipolar disorder.

Of course, this one case challenged our evaluation procedures and led to even more careful efforts being directed at the proper selection of potential STAPP candidates. One possible explanation of this case may be that the patient was seen at a time when her mood was at an even keel and she was able to get some help from her psychotherapy.

AN INTERNALIZED DIALOGUE

One of the most striking findings from our follow-up outcome studies has been the patients' descriptions of how they have utilized the new learning and problem solving skills which they have acquired during their STAPP to solve new psychological problems long after its termination. In the majority of the patients who had recovered we were able to hear descriptions of how such patients were utilizing what they had learned. In my book (Sifneos, 1972) I have given some samples of what patients had to say. Usually the follow-up evaluators were asked to insist on concrete examples from the patients in order to be satisfied that they were actually doing what they said and were not simply trying to please their evaluators.

I have called this finding an "internalized dialogue," where one part of the patient is asking the questions he thinks the therapist would have asked him if he were still in treatment, while the other part is attempting to associate or answer the questions. It is clear that this phenonemon points to an identification with a problem-solving therapist who is carried inside this patient's mind and whose task is to help him deal all alone with future emotional difficulties. In this way the patient feels immune and does not require further treatment, being able to rely on his own problem-solving abilities.

In a sense, then, one can argue that STAPP has become a truly preventive psychiatric treatment, and we are confident that it is indeed an appropriate therapy for our well-selected patients. It is clearly enjoyable for both therapist and patient, and it is a treatment which is fun to learn and to teach.

I have been asked repeatedly whether our STAPP patients could be treated successfully with any other kind of psychotherapy or even psychoanalysis. As far as other types of therapy are concerned, I have no way of knowing the answer. Anyone who is interested in treating STAPP candidates with a different treatment modality, and who can achieve similar results, should of course publish such findings. To my knowledge, no such outcome results have been made available. As far as psychoanalysis is concerned, I have no doubt that good results can be obtained. The question which remains is: Why should subjects be analyzed when they can achieve good results with STAPP, unless they are mental health professionals who wish to use the analytic experience for training purposes?

CHAPTER 14

STAPP for Older Patients and Individuals with Physical Symptomatology

A recent pleasant and unexpected discovery has been the finding that STAPP seems to be an effective treatment modality for elderly patients. Because our initial observations had been on young college students, we arrived at the erroneous conclusion that older patients would be somewhat rigid and unable to utilize a technique based on activity and focalization. As our experience grew, however, we cautiously decided to offer STAPP to elderly patients and were surprised to see that they seemed to benefit greatly from this treatment and that they were in many ways indistinguishable from our younger patients.

More recently I reviewed the STAPP of 17 patients 50 years and older. Nine were men and 8 were women. As might be expected, in 9 patients the focus of their therapy revolved around grief reactions over the loss of a loved one. What was more surprising, however, was the discovery that 8 elderly patients had clearly unresolved Oedipal problems with which they have lived for a long time and which they were able to overcome with the help of their therapists.

All patients were well educated and were psychologically minded.

They were sophisticated individuals who fulfilled all the STAPP criteria for selection and who agreed to work on a specified focus.

What was striking about these patients was their flexibility, their ability to establish a therapeutic alliance rapidly, and their ability to express positive feelings for their therapists early. Most of them also seemed to enjoy their lives, despite their psychological difficulties, and seemed to be future-oriented rather than looking back to their past experiences.

Here is an example of a STAPP session with an elderly patient:

A 72-year-old widow came to see me because of unresolved grief feelings about the death of her husband. The first few interviews had been taken up with her descriptions of her happy marriage and the good times she had had with her husband. It was on the fourth session that she described the hospital scene as she rushed to visit her husband, who had a myocardial infarction just one day before they were due to go on vacation, to which she was looking forward. She went on as follows:

PATIENT: I was packing when they called me with the news. I was shocked. I rushed to the hospital. I remember that the nurse would not allow me to visit Charles, but I begged them to let me, and I was able to see him and stay with him for a while. It was quite a shock. He looked so pale and so frightened. I held his hand, he smiled, and he seemed pleased that I was there, but soon after, he suggested that I should leave him. He said, "You look tired. Why don't you go and have something to eat in the cafeteria? I feel very tired and I want to sleep." I didn't want to go, but the nurse also came in the room at that point and she also urged me to leave. Reluctantly I got up. I waved to Charles. He smiled. When I returned later on in the afternoon the nurse told me that Charles had died a few minutes after I left. (*The patient looked sad. Her face had a tense expression.*)

THERAPIST: Of course, this is very difficult for you, but I do think that crying and expressing your grief is important and will help you overcome it.

PATIENT: But you see, doctor, I felt so guilty. I didn't cry.

THERAPIST: Why guilty?

PATIENT: Well, I left him and he died alone. I should have stayed with him. I should have been with him up to the last moment.

How could I go to the cafeteria to eat when he was dying at that moment?

THERAPIST: I think that you are too hard on yourself.

PATIENT: No! No! I deserve to suffer. I deserve to feel guilty.

THERAPIST: Yes, I think that you like to punish yourself, but the peculiar thing is that you punish yourself for the wrong reason.

PATIENT: Wrong reason? I don't know what you mean.

THERAPIST: Let's summarize what you said. You were looking forward to your vacation. You suddenly received the bad news that your husband had a heart attack. You were shocked, went to the hospital, and you visited him. It was an emotional encounter, but he soon asked you to go. You accepted reluctantly, but when you returned he had died. You did not cry, but you felt guilty because you were not with him during the last few moments of his life.

PATIENT: Yes. It is exactly as you say.

THERAPIST: Why did you think Charles wanted you to go away?

PATIENT: I don't know. Precisely why did he?

THERAPIST: Is it possible that he wanted to die alone, to die in dignity, and not to impose his death scene on you?

PATIENT: My God. I never thought of it. I never, never did. It is so obvious. It is the kind of thing that he would do. That was Charles and I never—it never crossed my mind. So stupid of me.

THERAPIST: There you go again, blaming yourself. Is the reason for punishing yourself the fact that Charles died at a very inconvenient time?

PATIENT: Oh, no. How can you say that!

THERAPIST: But it is true. You were going on vacation and you were looking forward to it.

PATIENT: There is something in what you say because when I was at the cafeteria I kept on thinking all about hotel reservations, plane tickets, cancellations, and so on.

THERAPIST: So?

PATIENT: (*pensive*): How could I when he was dying?

THERAPIST: That is why you feel guilty. Because of all those thoughts and not because you were not there during the last few minutes. I think that Charles knew, or was aware, that he was dying. This is a very private moment for all of us. He wanted to be alone, to die in dignity, and not to impose himself on his wife, whom he loved. He wanted to spare you the pain of seeing him die.

The therapist's recapitulation seems to have been successful. The patient returned the following week saying that she had been crying the whole time. She felt much better. Her unresolved grief reaction had been resolved.

It is usually acknowledged by internists and family physicians that a very large percentage of their patients complain of physical symptoms whose causes are usually psychological in nature. Because such complaints are usually treated only with reassurances or with tranquilizing medications, they persist, to the patient's dissatisfaction.

It was of interest to us to discover that several of our STAPP patients, in addition to the emotional difficulties which motivated them to seek psychiatric help, also complained of physical symptoms. There was no underlying pathology to account for their physical difficulties.

In our most recent study, which has already been described, 14 out of the 50 patients complained of physical symptoms. Thirteen were experimental ones and 1 was a control patient. Although at first they dissociated their physical difficulties from their psychological conflicts, it was clear to them after their evaluation that the two were connected.

These symptoms included the following: headache (5), diarrhea (1), insomnia (3), impotence (1), pain (1), tremors (2), anorexia (1), skin irritation (1), and cystitis (1).

Of seven patients who were scored as "recovered" after receiving STAPP, the physical symptoms disappeared in four and were much better in three. Of six patients rated as being "much better," the physical symptoms disappeared in 1, were much better in four, and were a "little better" in one. In the one patient whose STAPP was of no help and was rated as "unchanged," the physical symptoms persisted.

It can be concluded from these observations that this information should be made available to the physicians who are the first consulted by most patients for physical problems. If more of their appropriate patients are offered STAPP, they can be helped to overcome both their psychological and their physical symptoms.

CHAPTER 15

Epilogue

The development of short-term dynamic treatment modalities has revolutionized our thinking about psychotherapy in general. By specifying criteria for selection of appropriate candidates, by describing a variety of innovative techniques, and by investigating the outcome using scientific methods systematically, brief psychotherapies have succeeded in demonstrating their effectiveness and their value.

There is always, however, a caution which should be kept in mind with any kind of success story. One must not become overenthusiastic, develop a tendency to globalize, and apply these techniques indiscriminately to unsuitable patients. Furthermore, any attempts to modify these therapies as a result of political pressure or because of excessive demands for more service should always be resisted. Above and beyond these obvious considerations, however, the primary motivating force in developing short-term dynamic psychotherapy has been a dissatisfaction with the prevailing conformity to dogma and an enthusiasm for originality. These two qualities are the *sine qua non* of creativity. They should be cultivated at all costs so as to continue the momentum for the discovery of new therapies for more difficult patients.

Appendix I

The following case example of a 23-year-old female patient who received STAPP will be presented in detail not only to demonstrate to the reader the unfolding process of this kind of psychotherapy but also to illustrate the technical issues which have already been described in the previous chapters.

The patient was the youngest of three children. She was working as a secretary and came to the psychiatric clinic after she had had an abortion. She related that she had become pregnant by a boyfriend who treated her badly but for whom she felt considerable sexual attraction. She said that she wanted to understand the pattern of her behavior with men because she was anxious about it and was eager to learn why it invariably created difficulties for her.

Various details in language and style have been altered to protect the patient's confidentiality but in no way interfere with the truth about the nature and process of the treatment.

EVALUATION INTERVIEW

EVALUATOR: Please describe to me what bothers you most.
PATIENT: I have problems with men. I can't choose the right kind of a guy. I'm attracted to men who treat me badly, who care very little about me, and who want only sex. I don't know why I find such guys attractive. . . . . I get quite anxious about it.
EVALUATOR: Go on.

PATIENT: . . . I also have difficulty in getting along with people of my own age. I have trouble choosing friends.

EVALUATOR: When you say friends do you mean boy- or girlfriends?

PATIENT: Both.

EVALUATOR: What is the reason for this difficulty?

PATIENT (*Smiling*): Well, I'm a snob. I feel I'm unique. (*smiling*) Seriously. I would say that ever since I was a little girl I was with grown-ups. I enjoyed being with my parents.

EVALUATOR: Are you saying that your difficulty with people can be traced to your earlier experiences? (*The evaluator is testing the patient's self-inquisitiveness and psychological sophistication—two of the criteria for selection.*)

PATIENT: Yes. This is true, but it varied. . . .

EVALUATOR: In what way? (*The evaluator is encouraging the patient to pursue this subject and is rewarded.*)

PATIENT: I must say that I enjoyed much more being with my dad when I was little.

EVALUATOR: I see! We shall come to that point later, but let us now return to your difficulty with men, which is what brings you to the clinic. What actually did happen to make you decide to call for an appointment?

PATIENT: I was pregnant and I had an abortion. I got pregnant by this guy—his name is Jim—well, he's a nut. After my abortion I threw him out of my apartment and when he left I sat down and thought things out: "How did I get myself into such a mess? Why do I get attracted to such nuts?" I thought that the time had come to do something about it, so right there and then I called the clinic and made an appointment.

EVALUATOR: Could you describe to me your relationship with Jim?

PATIENT: There isn't much to say. We had sex together and it was enjoyable, but then he would get up and watch TV and pay no attention to me. I started getting fed up. Maybe by becoming pregnant I wanted to trap him. . . . No, no, it was more than that. Maybe I wanted a baby. I didn't want him. I wanted a baby . . . but then when I got pregnant and the reality hit me, I decided that I should have the abortion, and if I wanted a baby I should get it from someone else. So I went home and had my abortion.

EVALUATOR: Yet you say that you were attracted to Jim.

PATIENT: Sexually . . . yes, and I want to find out why I get attracted to guys like that, because it's happened several times before.

EVALUATOR: Did you ever get pregnant before?

PATIENT: No, this was the first and only time.

EVALUATOR: Do you have any other problems?

PATIENT: Of course, many problems. But the one with men is my greatest difficulty.

EVALUATOR: If we helped you understand it and solve it, will you be satisfied even if you have other problems which remain?

PATIENT: Yes, because all the others are minor ones compared to this one.

The evaluator, satisfied that the patient has a circumscribed chief complaint—the first criterion of selection for STAPP—is now ready to explore the patient's past history.

EVALUATOR: Now, let me ask you some questions about the past. How old are you?

PATIENT: Twenty-three.

EVALUATOR: Are your parents alive and well?

PATIENT: Yes.

EVALUATOR: How old are they?

PATIENT: My father is fifty-five and my mother is sixty.

EVALUATOR: I see . . . and do you have any brothers or sisters?

PATIENT: Yes, I have an older half brother and an older sister. My brother was from my mother's first marriage. Her first husband died and some years later she married my father.

EVALUATOR: How old are they?

PATIENT: My brother is forty and my sister is thirty-seven.

EVALUATOR: What is your earliest memory?

PATIENT: Earliest?

EVALUATOR: Yes, as far back as you can remember.

PATIENT: . . . Sitting with my father and mother and watching TV.

EVALUATOR: But watching TV is something that takes place later on, when one is older.

PATIENT: Oh, no, don't get me wrong. I wasn't watching TV. I was in my crib.

EVALUATOR: I see. Is this a pleasant memory?

PATIENT: Oh, yes, very much. So cozy . . . being with my parents (*smiling*).

EVALUATOR: So you loved your parents.

PATIENT: Very much . . . (*looking thoughtful*) Well, later on things changed, but when I was very young I loved my parents very much.

EVALUATOR: Both of them?

PATIENT: Yes, both.

EVALUATOR: What was your relation with your mother like?

PATIENT: At that early time it was fine. My mother and I used to spend a lot of time together. She taught me how to sew. She also taught me how to get along with adults. Later on it was difficult. My mother got sick with tuberculosis and was in a sanitarium off and on for several years. She also worked.

EVALUATOR: How old were you when she first went to the hospital?

PATIENT: I was six years old.

EVALUATOR: Were you your mother's favorite?

PATIENT: No, my older sister was. I was my daddy's favorite.

EVALUATOR: Tell me more about that.

PATIENT: Well, you see, my dad and I had great times together. We went on rides together.

EVALUATOR: Just the two of you?

PATIENT: Well, the times when it was only the two of us were the best. Well, when my mother was in the hospital, I cooked for my dad. I was very proud of it. I was like a "little wife."

EVALUATOR: A "little wife," eh?

PATIENT: Yes, I loved to take care of Dad. Those were the neatest times. (*smiling*) I'd do anything for him.

EVALUATOR: But what about your sister?

PATIENT: Oh, she was in college, so I took care of Dad. Actually, when my mother came back from the hospital I was glad to see her. But when she tried to tell me how to cook, I got mad because I knew how to do it . . . better than her.

EVALUATOR: Hm! So there was competition between the two of you.

PATIENT: At that time, yes, but when I was younger, and more recently, I had a good time with Mom. I do love her very much. Don't get me wrong.

EVALUATOR: I understand. Now, did you have any good friends?

PATIENT: Oh yes! In grammar school there was this girl, a neighbor of mine, we were inseparable. We are still good friends but we don't see each other now because she lives in Florida. But those early times, we had fun together.

EVALUATOR: Would you sacrifice anything for her?

PATIENT: What do you mean?

EVALUATOR: Well, I didn't put it well. What I mean is, can you give me an example of doing without something that you liked for the sake of your friendship with your friend?

PATIENT (*smiling*): Oh, yes, indeed! I had this Raggedy Ann doll that I loved. It was my favorite doll, but when Louise was sick in the hospital, I missed her so much. When she came back I was so glad to see her I gave her my doll.

EVALUATOR: That's what I had in mind. This is an excellent example. Okay, how were things at school?

PATIENT: So-so. I was not the best student but I did all right.

EVALUATOR: How did you get along with the teachers?

PATIENT: Very well. I was the teacher's pet.

EVALUATOR: Male or female teachers?

PATIENT: During grammar school they were all female.

EVALUATOR: How old were you when you had your first menstrual period?

PATIENT: I was twelve.

EVALUATOR: What was your reaction?

PATIENT: It was okay. I was prepared by my mother. I had also talked with my sister. I was glad to be a grown woman.

EVALUATOR: So you were proud of it?

PATIENT: Yes, I had looked forward to it.

EVALUATOR: Now, how was your early adolescence, the high school years?

PATIENT: Okay. I had a couple of friends. I had my first boyfriend— no big deal. It was then that I went to visit my sister. I was sixteen. After that time I started to be closer to my mother and I wasn't so close to Dad. During that visit all hell broke loose. My father didn't like my boyfriend. He made a scene. I stayed with my sister that summer. My parents also had a fight. The last two years of high school I was very close to my mother and when I graduated I was more interested in what she thought about than in what my father was interested in. It was a complete about-face.

EVALUATOR: Well, we must hear more about this, but first describe to me your college years.

PATIENT: There isn't much to say. I had a couple of boyfriends. They were nice but I lost interest in them. I had sex with one of them for the first time. It was I who seduced him because I was tired of being a virgin. I lost interest in him. It was around that time that I started being attracted to men who treated me badly. One guy, we had wonderful sex together but he used to come and wake me up in the middle of the night, have sex, and leave. It was whenever *he* wanted it. I resented it, but I was aroused and I gave in.

EVALUATOR: Did you enjoy sex with him?

PATIENT: Yes.

EVALUATOR: Did you have an orgasm?

PATIENT: Oh, yes, with these bad guys I always have orgasms; with the others, only sometimes.

EVALUATOR: With the "others" . . . you mean the nicer men?

PATIENT: Yes, exactly.

EVALUATOR: Now, what about your physical health?

PATIENT: Oh, I'm strong as an ox.

EVALUATOR: Has this always been the case?

PATIENT: Yes. I was always healthy, except for childhood diseases— measles, mumps, and once in a while a cold.

EVALUATOR: Fine. Now, what do you think is the cause of your difficulties with men?

PATIENT: I don't know, but it has something to do with the feelings I had for my father, which changed later on, as well as my feelings for my mother, which also changed. I tried to understand all this but I couldn't do it alone. I want to have someone give me a hand.

EVALUATOR: What do you expect from psychotherapy if we decide that it is indicated?

PATIENT: Well, I would like to understand all this, but I realize that it's going to be painful.

EVALUATOR: Are you prepared to do it despite the pain?

PATIENT: Yes.

EVALUATOR: Are you willing to make a sacrifice for this?

PATIENT: Well, I don't make too much money but I'm willing to pay for it, even if I have to miss some time at the office and have to make it up later on.

EVALUATOR: Okay, that's fine. Let's meet next week and go over all this once more. Now, I would like to have the interviews videotaped. Would it be all right with you? I'll explain to you what this is all about and you must read this informed consent form and sign it if you are willing.

PATIENT: Oh, it's okay by me.

The evaluator explained the purpose of videotaping, and the patient agreed and signed her permission, which was also countersigned.

The first videotaped interview was more or less a recapitulation of the evaluation interview. The decision to offer her STAPP was reached.

It should be clear from these interviews that the patient fulfilled all the criteria for STAPP. She clearly had an Oedipal problem, the exploration of which would become the therapeutic focus. It was also agreed that she would work hard with her therapist in order to disentangle her psychological problems, difficult as this might be.

FIRST THERAPY INTERVIEW

PATIENT: Well, as I have already told you, I have a problem with men. I seem to like sick men. I feel discouraged about it. I carry on and on in the same way, in the same pattern, and it's because I have a father hang-up.

THERAPIST: Can you give me an example?

PATIENT: Yes, there's Tony. He came over to my place on Monday late at night. He didn't call or anything. He stayed all night and we had intercourse. I felt sick because he's another nut. He's thirty years old. He doesn't treat me very well. He's demanding. My roommate gets very upset. He's nuts! He never takes me out or anything. He smokes grass and he drinks a lot. I'm tired of these guys. With Jim, for example, the one who made me pregnant, I threw him out. I don't want to see him again. I know I won't see Tony again. Yet, I slept with him. I want to break this pattern. I decided I wasn't going to do that again. I have another boyfriend, Mort. He's nice. He treats me very well. I was out with Mort and enjoyed myself. Yet, a few days later, despite all my resolutions, I sleep with Tony. He popped right in. I'm attracted to him. I enjoy his spontaneity. He has a lot of girlfriends.

THERAPIST: What about his having other girls. Do you find that attractive?

PATIENT: Well, he was going out with this other girl who wanted to get married and have a child. I had no one to go out with at that time, so I decided to rescue him.

THERAPIST: To rescue him?

PATIENT: Yes. I asked him to give her up, and if he did I promised to sleep with him.

THERAPIST: Now, let's try to figure out what is going on between you and Tony.

PATIENT: He meets all these interesting people (*smiling*) and there is this competition I have with Louise—that's the name of his ex-girlfriend. You see, I'm different. She smothered Tony with her dependence on him. He complained about it, so I decided I was going to be independent. I decided I was not going to smother him. I was going to be different.

THERAPIST: So your motivation was to separate them, to take Tony away from Louise?

PATIENT: Yes. Well, with Jim it was the same thing. He was married, then he was separated. His wife had a baby. There again I tried to be different from his wife. I tried to be independent. There was also another fellow when I was in high school. He had been going out with a girl for over a year, but I took him away from her. I cooked for him and I was faithful to him.

THERAPIST: So where does this pattern of behavior come from?

PATIENT: From Mother and Dad. My mother slept and I cooked breakfast for my dad. I had my father all to myself later on. I know that I competed with my mother for my dad, but when my mother and I had a fight, he always took my mother's side, but later on he would come to my room and apologize for his behavior. He said he did it for the sake of peace. And then there was my sister. Once I threw a bottle at her and I cut her foot. (*The patient proceeded to describe in some detail what happened, how her mother was upset but did not punish her. She took her sister to the hospital.*)

THERAPIST: So we have another conflict with a woman.

PATIENT: Well, it wasn't all over, because when my father came home, my mother told him what I had done, and he gave me quite a licking. He spanked my butt. I remember that it hurt. (*smiling*)

THERAPIST: But you are smiling.

PATIENT: Well, I liked the welts.

THERAPIST: So you enjoyed it?

PATIENT: Maybe. . . . There were those welts on my legs and on my bottom. I remember also another licking I got from my father, after my sister left for college. I don't remember any more spankings. When I was twelve or thirteen I was very close to my father, as I told you. I was proud to be grown up. I was becoming a grown-up lady, and I was accepted by my parents' friends. I enjoyed all this very much.

The therapist inquired about the patient's experiences in high school, which she described in some detail. She emphasized once more, however, that by the age of eighteen, she had become much closer to her mother. She described an episode at the airport as she was saying good-bye to her parents before she left for college. She had become upset when her mother didn't kiss her because her mother was taking her picture. She did not seem to appear to appreciate her father's attention to her at that time. She then related the following episode which had taken place a few years before her graduation from high school:

PATIENT: I had gone to visit my sister who was married by then. My parents also came to visit. I remember one morning my father had a black eye and he said that he had fallen down, but after my parents departed, my sister told me that my dad and her husband had gone out to a bar drinking. My father tried to pick up a prostitute, and when he went out with her, two men mugged him. When I heard that, I felt sick to my stomach. I felt really sick.

When she was asked about the details of this episode, she was reluctant to talk but associated to feeling sick after having intercourse with Tony.

THERAPIST: So it was the same feeling? The same reaction?

PATIENT: I felt sick . . . an icky feeling. I felt sick to my stomach, the exact same feeling after I had intercourse with Tony. . . .

The interview ended with the patient describing her fascination for prostitutes and emphasizing her admiration for their clothes.

This interview is typical of all STAPP patients. She talks rapidly, brings up valuable material about her competition with women in general and her mother in particular, and ends by drawing a parallel between her feelings for her father after the episode with the prostitute and her own reaction to Tony after having intercourse with him. There is very little necessary for the therapist to do under these circumstances since the material is flowing out so smoothly.

SECOND INTERVIEW

PATIENT: I've been thinking about Tony and Louise. She also wanted him to give her a baby. As I told you, I slept with him, but I was determined not to get pregnant. I wasn't going to ask him to give me a baby. I was going to be different. I was going to be above Louise.

THERAPIST: But you *did* get pregnant by Jim?

PATIENT: I wanted to give Jim a baby. You see, he had a child and he loved it so much. By having a baby I would have gotten a part of his life. At first, when I got pregnant, I wanted to keep the baby. I wasn't going to have an abortion.

THERAPIST: But you told me that you threw Jim out. Why did you do that?

PATIENT: If I had the baby, I wouldn't need Jim anymore.

THERAPIST: But that's a paradox, isn't it?

PATIENT: Well, it's the same thing with Jim as it is with Tony. They are both sick. Now with Mort—my current boyfriend—it's different. He's nice to me. He's like my other nice boyfriends. You see, I went with Tim for a year, but after a while I got tired of him. I lost interest. He was a nice, gentle country boy. We lived together like husband and wife, but I also kept my apartment. I also slept with other guys. I cooked for him.

THERAPIST: As you did with your father.

PATIENT (*ignoring this point*): He was very dependent on me. . . . I remember once during intercourse I called Tim "Dad." (*giggling nervously*) No, it happehed two or three times.

THERAPIST: So there's a clear-cut connection between your father and Tim.

PATIENT (*ignoring this statement*): Well, he was very dependent. He didn't like to be alone, and I disliked this attitude in him. Now, with my father it was different. I liked to be with him.

THERAPIST: What happened to make you get tired of Tim?

PATIENT: Well, I graduated from college. I had a car. I got a job. I had my apartment. I felt good about myself.

THERAPIST: What was your sexual relation with Tim like?

PATIENT: At first it was good. We had sex three or four times a day, but then it cooled down. Tim always wanted to talk. He had no experience, his lips were dry. I became bored with him. I got angry with him.

THERAPIST: Despite some differences, the nature of your relationship with Tim is in some way similar to the one you had with your father.

Again in a typical pattern of a good STAPP patient, she associated to the time when she lived with the family of a lawyer and took care of his young child. She again told of her antagonism for the lady of the house, whom she described as businesslike with not much feeling. She admitted wanting to give the lawyer, who was about her father's age, the attention that he did not receive from his wife. She also admitted wanting to give him the second child that his wife was unwilling to have.

Two additional aspects of this interview will be summarized. The first one had to do with the therapist's asking the patient if she used men so as to compete with women. The patient seemed to be somewhat interested in this, but she admitted that she was becoming disinterested in this neurotic battle with women. The second occurred at the end of this interview when the transference appeared in the form of a fantasy that she had in reference to the therapist. She thought that he would use the videotapes to expose her to others. Of course, as would be expected, the therapist dealt with this immediately, but because of the reality aspects involved with videotaping, he could not completely ignore them. Nevertheless, he was able to make the first parent-transference link. The patient associated spontaneously about her feelings for the therapist in a somewhat realistic way. She said that she felt somewhat threatened by him when he implied that the therapy was going to be hard work. She admitted having a fantasy that therapy might be easier with a woman or a younger man. The therapist pressed her to talk about this subject, and she admitted that she felt "intensely loyal" to women and much less so to men. Yet, at the same time, she admitted being stifled by women like her roommate. She also said that she craved to be free and independent. At this point the therapist was able to make the second parent-transference link by pointing out that again she seemed to have similar feelings for him as she had for her father.

Except for the technical maneuvers in the latter part of the interview, the patient seemed to continue working hard as she had done in the previous one, bringing up material in reference to relations with men and women in the present and connecting it with her relationship with her parents. She seemed to be staying within the Oedipal therapeutic focus—without requiring any assistance from her therapist.

THIRD INTERVIEW

The patient came to this interview wearing a very beautiful ensemble. She was well groomed and appeared to be in fine spirits.

PATIENT: I've been thinking about throwing Jim and Tony out after I slept with them. Yet there was a chance that I could get pregnant. Anyway, I didn't. Now, with Mort, it's different. He's nice. The other two are not.

THERAPIST: So getting pregnant and kicking the men out seem to be connected?

PATIENT: Getting pregnant is self-destructive, but maybe there's a wish to have a baby, and after I do I don't need the man anymore, so I get rid of him. The same thing happened to my sister. She got pregnant and then she got rid of her husband. He did his work and he wasn't needed anymore. His work was over—now, if I got my baby. . . .

THERAPIST: So maybe what you want is to have a baby by a different father.

PATIENT: A different father?

THERAPIST: Yes. Not the father who made you pregnant, but another father whom you would have liked to give you a baby, but who wouldn't, or he couldn't, or he was unwilling. . . .

PATIENT: I don't know.

THERAPIST: Now, this association of yours to what happened to your sister's husband is very interesting.

PATIENT: Maybe that's not what really happened.

THERAPIST: We are not interested at this point in what happened, but rather what counts is what goes on inside your head, how you interpret things.

PATIENT: Yes, I see.

THERAPIST: Okay. Now, let's look at all this from a different perspective. At what age did you learn about pregnancy?

PATIENT: In general?

THERAPIST: I mean about your being able to become pregnant and have a baby.

PATIENT: Around twelve.

THERAPIST: So at that time you realized that *you* could have a baby.

PATIENT: Well, maybe a little later. At twelve I had my period. Later I associated my period with pregnancy.

THERAPIST: Okay, if you were to have a baby, who would be the father of your baby?

PATIENT: I didn't think of anyone in particular. . . . Well, it could be the person that I married, such as Tim.

THERAPIST: Let's leave marriage out. In any case, you knew Tim when you were much older. I mean back then.

PATIENT: Yes, I see.

THERAPIST: Coming back to my question. If you wanted a baby and you didn't like the immediate father of that baby, the actual father, such as Jim and Tony, since you kicked them out, then is it possible that you wanted to have a baby by some kind of father that you liked but who could not give you a baby?

PATIENT: Some kind of a father! . . . I don't know. Can you repeat that question?

THERAPIST: Okay. You want a baby, but you don't like the person who gave you that baby, the man who made you pregnant, because you threw him out as you did with Jim.

PATIENT: Yeah.

THERAPIST: So if you wanted a baby and you didn't like the father, is it possible that you had in mind some other father by whom you would have liked to become pregnant? I was interested in that association you had about your sister and her husband. Now, at that time when you were twelve, thirteen, fourteen, did you think of anyone?

PATIENT: Well, I realized that I could have a baby when I had my period, as I told you.

THERAPIST: Exactly whom did you think of?

PATIENT: Whom did I think what?

THERAPIST: Whose baby?

PATIENT (*interrupting*): I don't know (*giggling*)—not my father!

THERAPIST: Who said anything about your father? (*laughing*)

PATIENT: Nobody.

THERAPIST: How did that thought come to mind?

PATIENT: Well, the only person I liked at that time was my father. Well, we're discussing all this father business, and I have the feeling that you're maneuvering (*gesticulating*) it all back to my father.

THERAPIST: Hold on! I am not maneuvering anything. I do, as you know, think that there was a special relationship between the two of you. Now, I am not trying to make you fit into anything—you know what the books say. What counts here are *your* thoughts. Now, if that thought about your father was in *your* mind, it is of great importance. So let's look at it.

PATIENT: I had no boyfriend at that time. I couldn't think of anyone else.

THERAPIST: Maybe you *didn't* think of anyone at that time. Now we don't have to stick to the age of twelve. Did you have the thought of being pregnant and having a baby when you were thirteen, fourteen? Who would the father be?

PATIENT: I didn't really think of who it could be.

THERAPIST: Well, is it possible that a young girl who acts "wife-like" with her father, who works for him and takes care of him, may have a thought about her father as the baby's father, and then dismiss it from her mind? What intrigues me was that you said, "Oh, no, no, it wasn't my father," and then you turn it all on me and imply that *I* am maneuvering to try to dig it out of you.

PATIENT (*giggling*): Oh, that was hostile! I didn't really. . . .

THERAPIST (*laughing*): It's all right. Now the question is, why didn't you?

PATIENT: Why did I?

THERAPIST: No, why *didn't* you?

PATIENT: I don't know . . . maybe I didn't want to. . . . (*looking pensive*) I didn't want to think of it.

THERAPIST: So!

PATIENT: Maybe that's why I pushed it out of my mind. Undoubtedly I did want my father to give me a baby.

THERAPIST: Are you saying that to please me? Now, tell me what is in your mind. You must take the responsibility of telling me what happened and not what you think is going to please me. Now, what comes to mind right now?

PATIENT: . . . Ah . . . okay. . . . I remember a dream that my father raped me. It was three or four years after I had my first period. I realized at that time that I could have a baby, at fifteen or sixteen. . . .

THERAPIST: Do you remember the details of that dream?

PATIENT: My mother was away and Dad raped me.

THERAPIST: What do you mean? What happened?

PATIENT (*giggling*): I don't like to think of that dream . . . well, he came into my room and had intercourse with me—my father, while my mother was away. I remember that dream distinctly. I felt so very guilty.

THERAPIST: So it was a nightmare?

PATIENT: I must have woke up after that dream. I hated myself for dreaming that kind of a dream.

THERAPIST: Now I did not know you then!

PATIENT: What?

THERAPIST: I didn't know you at that time, so I'm not responsible for that dream.

PATIENT (*laughing*): I'm not saying that you are.

THERAPIST: A few minutes ago you were saying exactly that.

PATIENT: That was hostile.

THERAPIST: No, no, I didn't mean it that way! That is not the point. I think what you did a few moments ago was to reject my question because you didn't like it. It is easier to make it my maneuvering—you know, what the psychiatrist wants to hear—than to look at the unpleasant realities of this dream. *You* had that dream. *You* had that thought about your father. After all, the dream points clearly to sexual aspects in reference to your father. You felt upset, you felt guilty. So at fifteen or so—we can pinpoint that in addition to your other "wifelike" duties in reference to your father—there were certain sexual thoughts which existed and which had to take the dream-path for their expression, when the mind is asleep.

PATIENT: . . . I had another dream shortly after. It was in the same home. I was raped by a stranger—not my father—but by someone whom I did not know. I remember that dream distinctly (*giggling*) . . . I remember all the details—the kitchen, the pots and pans that I used to cook, the road.

THERAPIST: Could you give me the details of what happened in that dream?

PATIENT: It was in my home and my kitchen. There was also the road where two of my girlfriends lived.

THERAPIST: Was it the house you lived in at the time?

PATIENT: Yes, it was my home. Well, a stranger came in, spread my legs apart. He couldn't rape me because . . it was the position of intercourse after some fondling around.

THERAPIST: Who was that unknown man?

PATIENT: He was older. I don't know who he was. All I can remember is the rape and the kitchen and the road. It was shortly after the dream that I had about my father. It was not as bad, however.

THERAPIST: So this dream was not as distasteful.

PATIENT: I remember it so distinctly! All the surroundings and that road.

THERAPIST: What about that road?

PATIENT: My mother used to drive me on that road taking me to school. It was a very familiar road.

THERAPIST: So your mother and your girlfriends are involved in this dream also. Then your mother is involved because this so-called rape took place in her kitchen.

PATIENT: *My* kitchen.

THERAPIST: What do you mean, *your* kitchen?

PATIENT: It was *my* kitchen.

THERAPIST: In reality it was your mother's kitchen, but in the dream it was yours.

PATIENT: . . . In reality . . . all right, I suppose so.

THERAPIST: So you took your mother's kitchen away from her.

PATIENT: Hm.

THERAPIST: Now, that man. What was his appearance? What did he wear?

PATIENT: A grubby appearance, I think . . . dirty, baggy pants and a T-shirt.

THERAPIST: Does he remind you of anyone you know?

PATIENT: . . . I don't know.

THERAPIST: No one in particular?

PATIENT: He was older. I was fifteen; he must have been about thirty.

THERAPIST: But now let us look at all this. First of all, it was not a rape.

PATIENT: Really?

THERAPIST: It was just getting ready to have intercourse.

PATIENT: Yes, he was just getting ready. It is true I couldn't remember having intercourse.

THERAPIST: But in the dream with your father there was intercourse.

PATIENT: Yes, it was real intercourse.

THERAPIST: Okay. Now, in this second dream, were you cooking?

PATIENT: I had all the pots and pans. I was getting dinner ready.

THERAPIST: You enjoy cooking, don't you?

PATIENT: Oh, yes, it's my favorite pastime. I love to cook. I used to cook a cake for my mother. My sister is also a good cook.

THERAPIST: So cooking dinner is an elaborate procedure that you enjoy.

PATIENT: I loved it. The best day in my life was once when I prepared dinner for my father and my uncle.

The patient proceeded to describe in detail her preparation of the meal, and her father's and uncle's teasing of her. She also mentioned that her mother was "a terrible cook," which the therapist laughingly acknowledged with the statement that he indeed had suspected so. At this point, the therapist attempted to get the patient's associations about the pleasures of cooking and producing a meal, and the planning of producing a baby. It was clear that, although the two might indeed have been connected, the discussion became intellectualized and bogged down. Belatedly the therapist changed tactics and asked her whether she had been dreaming recently, since the information about the two dreams had been so meaningful. The interview proceeded as follows:

PATIENT: Occasionally I do dream. When I was pregnant I dreamed a lot. I remember a dream about Tom, Jim's brother, who raped me. (*giggling*)

THERAPIST: He did, did he? What happened?

PATIENT: It was a few months ago and I remember the dream distinctly!

THERAPIST: So what happened with Tom in that dream?

PATIENT: Either he raped me or we slept together.

THERAPIST: I am struck again by the use of the word "rape." The word "rape" does not apply to the dream of the unknown man. Also, it does not apply in reference to Tom. You just said that he "either raped you or you slept together." Now the word "rape" involves the use of force by someone on another person who is unwilling. I am sure you know the exact meaning of the word "rape." So the question is, why do you use it incorrectly?

PATIENT: I wanted to sleep with Tom. I was attracted to him. I always wanted to have intercourse with Tom, but he was Jim's brother, and also I didn't want to sleep around as much, to be more selective, less promiscuous. Now, I said to him that I wanted to sleep with him, but that the only way he could get into my pants was by raping me. You know, we kidded around a lot. He's just as nuts as his brother, but he's nicer. We had some good laughs together about our mutual desires.

THERAPIST: That is quite intriguing! You decide that for various reasons you do not want to sleep with Tom, but it is all fine, you do sleep with him if he rapes you! You achieve what you want in this way, without taking the responsibility for it.

PATIENT: Yes.

THERAPIST: So in this rape situation with your father, with the unknown man, and now with Tom, it's the same story. They all have to be put in the position of raping you, because, if you take the responsibility of acknowledging your desire, it becomes very difficult and unpleasant for you. On the other hand, if you are raped by them then you are an innocent victim, and at the same time you achieve what you wanted, namely to satisfy your sexual desires, so you have your cake and eat it too!

PATIENT (*looking very apprehensive*): Yes . . hm, hm.

THERAPIST: Now, with Jim and Tony you were not unwilling, were you?

PATIENT: Oh, no. With them it was okay.

THERAPIST: So the use of the word "rape" is for only those who were prohibited, the fathers of your baby that were taboo! Yet all this does no good because you have to pay a huge price for it. You still have problems in your relations with women.

PATIENT: (*sighing*)

THERAPIST: You sigh!

PATIENT: . . . Well, I was thinking of my first sexual experience when I was nineteen. It was with a fellow I didn't particularly care about. I did it because I was tired of being a virgin. It was during my hippy period. I wasn't a very good hippy. I was play-acting. It was then that I went to see a social worker and was in treatment.

THERAPIST: You are running away from the subject that we were talking about, yet we must hear more about this phase of your life, too. However, the clock has come to your rescue. We must now stop.

This interview was presented in detail because it points to several technical aspects of STAPP. The therapist clearly stays within the Oedipal focus and asks anxiety-provoking questions repeatedly. He is rewarded, despite the patient's initial resistance and displacement onto him, with the priceless associations about the rape dream by the father. In this way, he is able to help the patient realize that her "wifelike" feelings for her father had pleasant and unpleasant sexual implications which are dealt with by the patient by her use of the word "rape." This defensive maneuver, however, is neurotic and is challenged by the therapist, although he realizes that the patient dislikes it and is anxious about it. Although he gets lost for a while in an unfruitful area, which is a technical mistake, he realizes it, and his question about the patient's current dreaming brings up another interesting dream about Tom. This enables the therapist to interpret and tie together her current feelings for men with her feelings for her father and the faceless unknown man, who is none other than her father in a more disguised form, increasingly camouflaged. Finally, the therapist points out that, although she gets what she wants by these neurotic maneuvers, she has to pay a very high price for it.

FOURTH INTERVIEW

When the patient arrived for her next session, she was dressed in a very flamboyant outfit with a very short skirt and looked radiant. She started the hour by emphasizing that she felt very well despite the fact that she remembered all the difficulties of the previous hour, which she called the "rape-dreams interview" and which she described as being very difficult. She said that she was perspiring all over when she left the office and went to meet her boyfriend Mort, who was waiting for her. She mentioned that she was eager to talk about a very interesting fantasy. It involved seeing somebody whom she mistook for Jim and she was puzzled about it because she knew that Jim was in Texas. Although she knew that this man was *not* Jim, she was nevertheless obsessed with the idea that it *was* Jim. She attributed to him superhuman and magical powers. She associated further to a statement that Jim had made when they were going out together, that he had the power to make all his women do whatever he wanted them to do. For example, he told her that he could make her be a prostitute and work for him. The therapist immediately asked her whether Jim's statement about her becoming a prostitute and her subsequent fascination for prostitution were connected. She seemed to be resistant at this point, but the therapist persisted and reminded her of the episode between her father and the prostitute, when her father was mugged. She said that she saw no connection between the two situations. At this point the therapist made the following anxiety-provoking confrontation:

THERAPIST: Now what would happen if you had become one of Jim's prostitutes and met your father at the bar?
PATIENT (*giggling*): Oh! No! No! Never!

Soon after this exchange, however, the patient's good spirits, which had predominated up to that point, changed dramatically. She again described her horror when she heard about the episode between her father and the prostitute, but she also emphasized her fascination for prostitutes particularly because they had the money to buy beautiful clothes. She also remembered having felt very upset when a man of her father's age had propositioned her. Her reaction was "My God, I could be his daughter!" Finally, she started to accuse her father of being "rotten," because if he could have intercourse with a prostitute, then he could sleep with her. And then, bursting into tears, she explained,

PATIENT: I hate my father and I hate me too.

Although the emphasis had been more on blaming her father, the therapist decided not to remind her of her own dreams, her own sexual feelings for her father, and her own responsibility for these feelings, because he felt that she showed so much feeling during this exchange that it might have been almost cruel at this point to make her feel worse. Thus, as has been emphasized, STAPP is not anxiety-provoking all the time, and on many occasions the therapist may decide to be quite supportive of the patient, particularly when the patient is working hard and is experiencing painful feelings, as the patient had been during the above-mentioned exchange. Since one of the issues had been the patient's fascination for clothes, the therapist decided to pay attention to this and to comment on the patient's appearance. This produced a marked change in her. She talked in glowing terms about clothes in general and about her own in particular. She said that she was proud of her appearance the day of the interview: "I woke up feeling fine . . . I'm dressed up to parade all over town and to come for my session and to be seen by anyone who might be interested in me!" This brought the positive transference into the open. It was discussed at length for the balance of the interview. Thus the therapist was able to make several important transference interpretations which the patient acknowledged.

At the end of the hour, the therapist reminded her that he would be away the following week and would see her at the regular time two weeks hence. The patient was flustered by this, asked what the date would be, and appeared downcast as she was leaving the office.

FIFTH INTERVIEW

As was predicted, the patient came for this interview looking somewhat unkempt and not very well groomed in comparison to the previous two sessions. She was silent and generally seemed to be withdrawn and subdued. She talked about the therapist's being interested in other important matters and associated this to her father's agreeing with her mother when her mother punished her, but then coming to her room and apologizing to her. The obvious parent-transference links were made repeatedly during this interview, but the therapist, possibly because he was a bit taken aback by the strength of the patient's reaction to the cancellation of the previous interview, tended to become more talkative, more intellectualized, and somewhat apologetic. The patient took advantage of this and talked in the following way:

PATIENT: When I left this office I felt forsaken. I took to the subway and I sat next to an old man who looked very sad. I felt sorry for him and I felt sorry for myself. I burst into tears and I cried all the way back to my home.

THERAPIST: So you felt that I let you down?

PATIENT: Yes. I felt that nobody loved me.

THERAPIST: Why all this "poor me" attitude?

PATIENT: Well, you could have been more supportive, more helpful.

THERAPIST: So you had some strong feelings about me. Now what about all this?

PATIENT: You were going to be busy doing other more important things, but you could have paid a little more attention to me.

THERAPIST: So as I said, you felt that I let you down. I seem to have disappointed you in the same way that your father disappointed you.

PATIENT: Exactly. I thought that maybe you tricked me, just to see what my reaction was going to be.

THERAPIST: No, I do not trick people.

PATIENT: Well, I've been thinking about my feelings for you. I asked myself all week whether I'm attracted to you sexually. I am interested in you. I'm intrigued by your faint English accent, but finally I decided that I was annoyed at you.

THERAPIST: I am glad that you bring all these feelings into the open. Now, some of these feelings are similar to feelings that you had for your father, as we have already seen before as well as earlier today. In addition, there are some realistic feelings that you have for me personally which are difficult. Now, you could have mentioned that you felt let down during the interview. If you felt sad and disappointed, it was important to bring it up as you did.

The interview went on for a while along these lines, with the therapist attempting to support the patient's self-esteem. Toward the end of the hour the patient started to work hard again. She associated again to her love for clothes and said that she always felt embarrassed and guilty whenever she bought an expensive dress.

The discussion about clothes led her to talk about her mother, who she felt disapproved of her being extravagant. The therapist emphasized that this was probably more the patient's problem because of her guilt feelings in reference to her attraction for her father, the episode about the prostitute, her "wifelike" activities, and so on. Thus a golden opportunity was offered to the therapist to recapitulate and tie together all the work that had been done so far during the first five interviews of the patient's therapy. At the end of the hour, the patient stated emphatically that she was glad to work on all these difficult subjects because she did not want to have a bad relationship with her mother, whom she loved, as a result of her feelings for her father, who did not deserve all her attention.

One could say, at this point, that the therapy had reached a crossroad. The work on her feelings for her father and men in general, as well as her therapist in the transference, had almost been completed. Now the more difficult task that remained was to clarify the impact such feelings had on her relation with women in general and with her mother in particular. The next few interviews played a crucial role in the transition from one area to another. Although this is contrary to what happens with female patients, it is speculated that, if she had a female therapist, the task would be even more difficult.

SIXTH INTERVIEW

It was clear that peace had been established between the patient and her therapist. She again came for her session attractively attired and looking very well groomed.

PATIENT: I've been thinking a lot about last week's session. Many of the things that you said went over my head. There was, however, the problem of being dressed up, having something to do with

my mother, and of course the wish to be a prostitute and that
rape dream all associated with my father. I had many thoughts.

THERAPIST: So, what do you think about all this?

PATIENT: Well, I bumbled my session last week. I did that because
you let me out the previous week. I pulled a trick on you.

THERAPIST: Were you aware of it at the time, during the interview?

PATIENT: No. I was not aware that I was angry at you at first, because you did not see me. I was aware of my anger at my father.
Also the notion of wanting to be a prostitute for him, which we
had discussed before, upset me very much. I felt that I wanted to
clear up all this stuff.

THERAPIST: Yes, but what you were most upset about was that I
didn't give you an extra hour.

PATIENT: Yes, that's true.

THERAPIST: Is it possible that there was something special about that
hour?

PATIENT: Well, I tricked you and I tricked myself. I told you all
about my fears, being very upset and all that. I didn't ask for an
extra hour, but I've been thinking a lot about it. For example, I've
been thinking of writing to ask you to extend the hour to fifty
minutes instead of the forty-five minutes that we now have. I
thought of having two sessions a week to speed things up. Also, I
wanted to ask you for another day, which would be more convenient for me. As you said last time, I have the right to ask.

THERAPIST: Of course.

PATIENT: Yet I don't ask.

THERAPIST: Now, going back to your saying that you tricked me.
Did you realistically want to have an extra hour, or did you simply want to manipulate me because you were angry? Now, if you
say you were angry, the question is, what were you angry about?
Is it possible that there was something special about that hour?
Now let's try to recapitulate what happened. You were feeling
fine, you were all dressed up, you expected to have a good hour,
a good time, but you did not. It was a difficult hour. You were in
tears, and then I told you that there was not going to be an extra
hour. Was this a letdown followed by anger?

PATIENT: I was very happy. I didn't believe that you were not going
to offer me another appointment.

THERAPIST: So you were not angry at me initially, as you say and as we know. You were angry only after you found out that I was not going to offer you another appointment. Now, you had two reactions. You felt forsaken and sad and you cried in the subway, but then when you came for your session last week you were angry.

PATIENT: I know that. I was aware of it during the interview. It was a crummy session.

THERAPIST: So you see that we must analyze what happens between us here, because if we can understand what goes on between you and me, we may be able to understand better your behavior outside of this office, with other people. So your expectations were not fulfilled and you had a letdown. Now, does that remind you of anything?

PATIENT: Yes. I had expectations for a fun weekend with Mort. I was looking forward to seeing him for two whole days. It was my birthday. You know what? He came late, and he hadn't even picked the restaurant where we were going to go . . . and then my dad. . . .

THERAPIST: Go on.

PATIENT: Nothing definite just now . . . .

THERAPIST: You said, "my dad . . . ."

PATIENT: Well, there was my high school prom after which I expected my parents were going to take me out for dinner, but they didn't. I expect a lot.

THERAPIST: . . . Nothing else comes to mind? For example, when you were younger, when you were a child, were you sensitive as a child?

The therapist is aware that there might be some important memory likely to come up, judging from the patient's facial expressions. She seemed to have something in mind, but either it was not very clear or she was resisting, so he persisted in his encouragement of her. He tried to move from the transference feelings, which were clarified in the early part of the interview, to feelings about her father in her childhood. What follows proves that he was on the right track:

PATIENT: I do remember Sundays. Sundays were very special days for me. Dad and I were always together. We would watch TV. I would prepare his drink. Sundays with a man are very special.

(*giggles*) I always looked forward to Sundays. I had high expectations, but if my father had to go to some meeting, I had a big letdown. My Sunday was ruined.

THERAPIST: When was all this?

PATIENT: When I was . . . well, up to the age of thirteen.

THERAPIST: Did it last after that?

PATIENT (*interrupting*): Before? I didn't care what I watched on TV—car races, or any old thing. I didn't care what I was watching.

THERAPIST: But what happened after you matured, after you developed physically?

PATIENT: (*laughing*)

THERAPIST: Why do you laugh?

PATIENT: (*giggling*)

THERAPIST: Come on, what's going on?

PATIENT (*continuing to giggle*): There we go again! This sexual attraction for my father. I was very affectionate with my father at that time.

THERAPIST: Let's look at all this. Now, if you didn't care what you were watching on TV, what counted was the interaction with your father, your being together. You said, "My Sunday was ruined when he went away." What about all this?

PATIENT: You mean why my Sunday was ruined?

THERAPIST: No, I understand why it was ruined. What I'm interested to know was what thoughts did you have when you were sitting *next* to your father on Sundays when you *weren't* watching TV.

PATIENT: What thoughts when he disappointed me? (*Clearly she is resisting the implication of the therapist's question.*)

THERAPIST: No, no. What thoughts raced through your head when you *were* together?

PATIENT (*smiling*): Oh . . . I was sitting there. I was a "little wife," as we discussed, while my mother was away.

THERAPIST: This is a neat way to globalize. (*What the therapist does here is try to help the patient specify her fantasies and thoughts more concretely and not to use headlines to globalize so as to run away from the anxiety-provoking material. This is a typical STAPP technical maneuver.*) You say "little wife" or "I had a sexual attraction for my father" and so on. These are headlines. They don't tell us what it means to be a "little wife." The way you put it helps you avoid thinking about and talking about the details, because those details are very unpleasant, such as the rape dream with your father. Now, can you tell me what your thoughts were, what your fantasies were of being a "little wife" to your father?

PATIENT: Well, it was my father and me, my father and I. Sometimes I'd sit close to him. It was cozy and warm. I'd kiss him good night, I'd sit on the arm of his chair. I kept him cozy and comfortable.

THERAPIST: How did you feel physically about all that?

PATIENT: Probably (giggling) . . . a little turned on, I don't know.

THERAPIST: Now, what do you mean?

PATIENT: As I said, we were very affectionate with each other . . . .

THERAPIST: Meaning?

PATIENT: I'd snuggle up to him. I'd kiss him good night. Even until I was twelve years old. I'd go into the bathroom and wash my father's back when he was in the tub.

THERAPIST: What were your thoughts when you were washing your father's back when he was in the tub?

PATIENT: Well . . . (giggling) I couldn't believe his genitals. (giggling)

THERAPIST: What do you mean by that? "You couldn't believe," you say.

PATIENT: They were so large, with deep blue veins on his testicles and his penis.

THERAPIST: You say you couldn't believe what you were looking at? What does that mean? Were you afraid?

PATIENT: Well, it was not an attractive sight.

THERAPIST: Yes . . . .

PATIENT: . . . And (looking very thoughtful) . . . I was sort of afraid.

THERAPIST: There is no warm feeling in all this. Look at it this way: you talked about something very positive between you and your father a few minutes ago—the TV, the drink, the kisses—but following these very positive memories something else popped into your mind which was obviously not as pleasant, something unattractive and a bit scary. Now, did you have any other thoughts about all this?

PATIENT: Ah—

THERAPIST (*interrupting*): Now, all this was going on before or after the rape dream with your father?

PATIENT: I had the dream afterward, when I was thirteen or fourteen. This was . . . .

THERAPIST: So seeing your father's genitals in the bathtub occurred before the dream.

PATIENT: Yes, definitely before. It was before my going to visit my sister . . . . (*looking very apprehensive*)

THERAPIST: I know that all this is difficult.

PATIENT: Yes. (*giggling nervously*)

THERAPIST: You know the reason we're going into all this in so much detail is because the sequence of all these events, pleasant and unpleasant, is very important. Now, shall we try to disentangle all this a bit?

PATIENT: Hm.

THERAPIST: Okay. Now, the dream occurred after the age of twelve, somewhere between thirteen and fifteen. The good times, the TV and all that, was all before twelve, and the bathtub episode went on until the age of twelve. Is that correct?

PATIENT: Yes, definitely, also likely, I went to visit my sister when I was fourteen.

THERAPIST: Was the dream, the rape dream, before that visit?

PATIENT: Positively before.

THERAPIST: So it was a bit earlier. But the bathtub episode, which was unpleasant, occurred between the good times, the TV times, and the two so-called rape dreams. Now, how much do you think the bathtub episode influenced you? Did it also have something to do with those dreams?

PATIENT: Seeing his genitals?

THERAPIST: Had you ever seen any male genitals before that time?

PATIENT: No other than my father's.

THERAPIST: Hadn't you seen any little boys before?

PATIENT: Oh, yes, little boys. Yes.

THERAPIST: Did you play with little boys?

PATIENT: Oh, yes. There was this little kid—we played doctor. I was fascinated by his genitals.

THERAPIST: Hm!

PATIENT: Yes, I was.

THERAPIST: How old were you?

PATIENT: Eight at the very latest.

THERAPIST: What fascinated you?

PATIENT: Well . . . his penis . . . (*silent for a long time*) . . . Well, it was the size . . . the shape . . . the feel of it. His sister was there. I was older than the both of them.

THERAPIST: You were "fascinated by" versus "frightened by." Isn't that interesting?

PATIENT: You see, my father was old, versus (*giggle*) . . . you know. He was . . . well, his genitals were bigger (*giggles*), fluffy . . . the kid's were smaller, smoother . . . kind of tight . . . .

THERAPIST: Hm . . . It's clear that there were very different reactions to those two situations. Now with the little boy, when you were eight, was that the first time that you had seen male genitals?

PATIENT: I'm quite sure it was . . . no! No, when I was about six my dad, my sister, and I took baths together. I remember the house we were living in at that time . . . so I'd seen my dad before I'd seen the little kid.

THERAPIST: Did you remember noticing your father's genitals at that earlier time?

PATIENT: I can't remember exactly, but I do remember noticing his genitals. I don't remember any fear or envy. I don't . . . but I did notice them—definitely.

THERAPIST: So you noticed that you and your sister were different from your father.

PATIENT: Yes, I knew that.

THERAPIST: Well, now, what was your reaction?

PATIENT: I don't remember clearly.

THERAPIST: So you just noticed that you were different, that was all?

PATIENT: . . . I was fascinated. I snuck a few extra looks. . . .

THERAPIST: Aren't you intrigued by what you said? You were fascinated when you noticed your father's genitals when you and your sister took a bath with him. You were six years old. You were fascinated, when you played doctor, by the little boy's penis when you were eight. Now, when you saw the same sight at about twelve, namely, your father in the tub, you were frightened. No fascination, but rather you emphasized how unattractive the whole thing was. Now, in six years I don't think that your father had changed in any way. So the change was in you.

PATIENT (*with much emphasis*): Well, at twelve I knew what the genitals were for.

THERAPIST: What about that?

PATIENT: Well, I could hear my parents having intercourse.

THERAPIST: Can you tell me something about this?

PATIENT: That threw me . . . . It was unfair. The walls were paper thin. I was physically turned on. I remember that feeling distinctly! I was very turned on.

THERAPIST: Whenever you use the word "distinctly" I'm convinced that it is so.

PATIENT: I also felt angry. I felt very uncomfortable when I saw my mother the next day. It was unpleasant to be around my mother. I thought that my father hurt my mother during intercourse.

THERAPIST: Now, how old were you when all this was happening?

PATIENT: From eleven on. I heard them having intercourse when I was twelve or thirteen.

THERAPIST: So it's all around that same time. Now, how did you know that they were having intercourse?

PATIENT: I knew.

THERAPIST: How did you know?

PATIENT: Don't kids just know?

THERAPIST: What I'm interested in is, how did *you* find out, because you didn't know between the ages of six to eight and because you were fascinated without being horrified.

PATIENT: I knew after that, between eight and twelve. I heard about it in school. I played doctor also with other girls. I also had discovered that my clitoris was a very sensitive part of me.

THERAPIST: Playing doctor. Now, what did that amount to?

PATIENT: We examined each other. We touched each other. It felt good. It was all girls. I didn't know any boys in that time. The only boy I knew was that little kid I told you about a few years before. Well, there was also some talk about my cousin trying to rape my sister. I didn't know what happened exactly, but there was a lot of talk and hush-hush.

THERAPIST: So, did you have any other thoughts at the time? We know that you had discovered that you could derive pleasure from your own genitals.

PATIENT: Oh . . . wait a minute.

THERAPIST: Go on. What did come to mind?

PATIENT: When I was six or seven, four marines came looking for my sister. I went out to see what it was. I was wearing my pajamas. One of the guys sat me on his lap. I wore no underclothes. He felt me all over.

THERAPIST: Yes. But still at eight you weren't particularly scared. Now, let's get back to the word "fascination"—what does that imply? What were you fascinated by?

PATIENT: . . . Sort of like . . . I don't believe what I'm seeing is true.

THERAPIST: Why?

PATIENT: Why? Why I was fascinated?

THERAPIST: No, rather why what you saw was not true?

PATIENT: Because it was so different from what I had.

THERAPIST: Precisely.

PATIENT (*giggling*): You!

THERAPIST: So you were aware of the differences.

PATIENT: When I took a bath with my father, I was amazed that someone would be so different.

THERAPIST: Did the thought occur to you to ask why you were the way you were or why he was that way?

PATIENT: . . . Let me see. Did I ask my mother? No. After I saw the little boy I examined myself closely. I remember that distinctly! (*giggles*)

THERAPIST: . . . And. . . .

PATIENT: I didn't have a penis. . . . (*blushing*)

THERAPIST: What is the feeling that you're experiencing right now?

PATIENT: . . . I don't like the thought that I was ever envious of any man's genitals. Oh! . . . I don't like that thought!

THERAPIST: Did that thought occur to you?

PATIENT: Probably. Well, also I know what the books say.

THERAPIST: Let's forget what the books say, or what is fashionable, or what the psychiatrists are supposed to say. What we are interested in understanding here are *your* thoughts, *your* experiences. What happened to you.

PATIENT: Well, I can't arrive at any definite conclusions. I'm not sure that I have the evidence that I felt envious. What I did was to look at myself to see if there was one hanging around that I hadn't noticed before.

THERAPIST: The fact that you had to go and look was that the fascination which you experienced gave rise to some sort of a thought which now motivated you to look at yourself more carefully.

PATIENT: Yes.

THERAPIST: It seems that that thought is lost.

PATIENT: You mean whether I was disappointed or not?

THERAPIST: Not necessarily that you were disappointed or not. I'm interested in the feeling and in the thought that you had.

PATIENT: I don't remember.

THERAPIST: After you looked at yourself, and examined yourself carefully, did you look at the little boy again?

PATIENT: No . . . I felt a little embarrassed.

THERAPIST: So the games that you played together stopped after that.

PATIENT: Yes, they did with the little boy, but not with the girls.

THERAPIST: Yes, but little girls were like you. I meant with boys. So the next time that you looked at male genitals again was when you were twelve, when you washed your father's back again.

PATIENT: Yes. I saw nothing between eight and twelve.

THERAPIST: Now, let's recapitulate once more where we are. You were fascinated between the ages of six and eight looking at your father's and the little boy's genitals, which looked very different, yet the fascination was the same. Furthermore, you discovered that you derived pleasure from your own genitals and that you were different. You examined yourself carefully but you don't remember any thoughts or feelings about that—no disappointment, no envy, no pride. You also discover that there is nothing like the little boy's penis in you down there. After that you feel a bit embarrassed. You immediately stop playing with the little boy. You play with other little girls. From then on you don't play with any boys and you don't see any male genitals. You are sure about that? I mean until the age of twelve when you saw your father's again?

PATIENT: Yes, I didn't. No other little boys. I'm sure. Then I saw my father's in the tub at twelve or thirteen.

THERAPIST: Your reaction at that time was entirely different. "Ugly," "unattractive," and there is also some fear. Now, your father had not changed very much in six years.

PATIENT: No.

THERAPIST: So the change was in you, and this was due to two things which you learned about. The first one was that you looked at yourself and found out that you were different from the little boy. You also heard something about intercourse at school; not from what you heard about your parents, that was later on. I think what happened to you at twelve when you saw your father again was that you had a delayed reaction from the episode with the little boy and from looking at yourself. It was clear at twelve that you didn't want to have such an ugly, unattractive organ.

PATIENT: Why after such a long time?

THERAPIST: You discovered that you did not have something hanging there. Maybe you thought that you should have, or that you lost it if it were there. Whatever you thought, it was clear you exaggerated the ugliness of what you saw four years later, veins and all that. So to reassure yourself for not having something, you felt embarrassed. You decided that you didn't want to have such an ugly thing. You decided that you were much better the way you were, like the other little girls, and furthermore, there was pleasure out of what you had.

PATIENT: When my mother and father had intercourse, my mother always sounded as if she were in pain. She had her orgasm, I guess. . . .

THERAPIST: That was later on, when you were fourteen or fifteen.

PATIENT: Yes . . . (smiling) I'm glad to be a woman.

THERAPIST: Of course! Of course you're glad to be a woman!

PATIENT: I am!

THERAPIST: As you can see, it's helpful for us to know the sequence of events, as well as all the details which are involved, as difficult as it may be at times. Now. . . .

(The patient gets up and is leaving the office.)

THERAPIST: I haven't even mentioned that the time is up and you're already halfway out of the room. Why are you running away so fast?

PATIENT: I don't want to overextend the interview.

THERAPIST: Hm. Okay! I'll see you and we'll talk about all this next week.

This interview is obviously very anxiety-provoking. The therapist has tried in a very careful way to put together the information provided him by the patient who, by virtue of her anxiety, tries to resist.

Although it is possible that his interpretations may be

challenged, what counts is the painstaking quality of amassing the data provided to the therapist by the patient, and sorting it out in a step-by-step way, paying special attention to the sequence and the timing. This gives the patient a completely different picture of what happened. It is like a jigsaw puzzle in which all the bits and parts are pieced together during the interview. This is a vital technical part of STAPP which has already been referred to as "problem solving."

From our follow-up work it appears that this technique constitutes one of the most useful learning experiences for the patient because it can be utilized by him effectively a long time after the treatment has been terminated.

It should be emphasized that despite the painful feelings experienced by the patient, her pride in being a woman was strongly emphasized by her, as well as by the therapist, in the latter part of the interview.

The therapist thought that the examination and understanding of the patient's relations with men had been completed. Now her relations with women had to be scrutinized and understood. The questions to be answered were: What would all the women, with her mother leading the group, do to retaliate for having been defeated by the patient and having lost their men? And how would the patient manage to appease all these angry women? The next two interviews provide the answers to these questions.

SEVENTH INTERVIEW

The patient opened the seventh interview by stating that despite the difficulty of the previous session, she was happy with it because she understood a lot about herself. As evidence of this she mentioned that she had remembered several episodes which had occurred with her boyfriend Tim, whom she had on occasion called "Daddy" while she was having intercourse with him (she also mentioned that she dropped him after a while because she grew bored of his dependence on her).

The therapist said that this aspect of her behavior had already been discussed between them previously, but he emphasized that it had not been clear what had actually made her become disinterested in her various boyfriends.

The patient went on to mention that what she had remembered during the past week had been a special memory. It appears that on occasions while she was having intercourse with Tim she had the fantasy that she had detached his penis from him and possessed it herself. In addition she remembered that she had referred to his penis as her own. She said that she did not know why she had done all this, or why the memory popped into her mind, but she seemed to have attributed it to the discussion of the previous hour. Nevertheless, she emphasized that as a result of the last session she had felt very proud of being a woman. She gave as an example the fact that Mort had recently admired her figure and had paid her compliments. She also said that several people had liked her clothes. What she emphasized most, however, was her own pride in herself and her own feeling of well-being. At this point the therapist recapitulated the issues that were discussed during the previous hour and he went on:

THERAPIST: Now, can we go back to this episode with Tim? What are the thoughts that come to mind?

PATIENT: Well, you see he was very dependent. He would run around after me all the time. He would ask me what to do. He always wanted something from me. He was very weak.

THERAPIST: But you say that on occasions you called him "Daddy." Isn't that so?

PATIENT: Yes, I did.

THERAPIST: So there is a connection between your boyfriend Tim and your father in your own mind.

PATIENT: Yes. I took a lot from Dad. He took a lot from me.

THERAPIST: In what way?

PATIENT: They were all weak. You see, I could get anything I wanted from all of them. They were dependent on me, as my father was for his drink or his supper. I could use them. I could manipulate them both.

THERAPIST: What about all this?

PATIENT: When I said "my penis," did I take it away from them just for my own use?

THERAPIST: Did you?

PATIENT: Do I want to emasculate men? (looking very thoughtful and making a grimace) Do I? For example, last time when you were talking at the end of the hour, I cut you off. I got up and left. I ran away. You were trying to explain something to me. Was I trying to emasculate you?

THERAPIST: A very good question. What do you think?

PATIENT: . . . Well! . . . If I emasculate you, I take all the pressure that you were exerting on me off my back.

THERAPIST: Okay, can we try to disentangle all this?

PATIENT: Yes. If I emasculate you, not only do I take the pressure off, but I also take away your professional power, your professional ability from you. You become useless to me.

THERAPIST: So we have a parallel here between your wishes for your boyfriend, for your father, and for me.

PATIENT: Yet, I love men. (*with much feeling*) I have a good time with men, as I did with my father.

THERAPIST: I know, but you also want to use them. Now, what about the bad men to whom you are attracted?

PATIENT: I used to be.

THERAPIST: Are you saying that you are not anymore?

PATIENT (*ignoring the question*): Well, I used their penises. I became pregnant and then I discarded them. They were useless.

THERAPIST: Does this apply to Mort?

PATIENT: I have a good relation with Mort. I like him. I was even thinking of getting married to him. It would be neat, but deep inside I don't want to marry him. I don't want to marry anybody right now unless I clear all this up. I'm not attracted to bad men anymore.

THERAPIST: Hm.

The patient continued to talk at length about various experiences she had had with several of her boyfriends, and described her feelings about them. It appears that invariably she became tired and bored and she would drop them. With two men she said that she felt disgusted, she became intolerant, and finally she moved away from them. She went on as follows:

PATIENT: Now, I foresee that I may do the same thing with Mort. Yet I love Mort as I loved my father.

THERAPIST: So this occurs more with people whom you love?

PATIENT: Yes, because with the others, the bad ones, I don't care so much what happens to them afterward, but I do care what happens to men I love. This emasculation tendency in me bothers me very much. I want to discuss it and to understand it. Why do I do it? I love being a woman and I do want to have a good relation with a man, to get married, and to have a family. This emasculation thing worries me and if I do it to Mort, it will be too bad.

THERAPIST: So there is excitement and good feeling at first, as you now have for Mort and as you had for your father; and then there is the need to move away, disgusted by them.

PATIENT: Hm. Yes . . . (looking thoughtful)

THERAPIST: So you are first "fascinated" and then "disgusted."

PATIENT: . . . Gee . . . hm . . . you're a genius! (smiling)

THERAPIST: No compliments, please. Let's find out why.

What is most striking in this hour is the patient's motivation to change. She brings up a very unpleasant thought which she admits bothers her very much. Nevertheless, she sticks to it, raises important questions in reference to the past, as well as the transference, and gives the opportunity to the therapist to make a parent-transference link interpretation. In addition, a golden opportunity is offered to him to tie the material that emerged from the previous interview with her need to emasculate men.

It is obvious that the therapy has reached its zenith, and the painful feelings which emerged will have to be dealt with in one way or another. One could speculate at this point what might happen in the following hour. Would she continue to work hard? Would she act out in some way? Would she regress somewhat to avoid the pain? In any case, the therapist must be ready to deal with any eventuality.

EIGHTH INTERVIEW

The patient came for her interview on time, but again, as in the fifth interview, she was somewhat unkempt, her hair pulled back, her clothes somewhat ill fitting. She seemed to be tired and somewhat withdrawn.

PATIENT: I had the feeling I'd be sick so as not to have to come today.

THERAPIST: Does it have to do with last week's session?

PATIENT: I don't know. . . . Well, yes. There's this pattern that we talked about and I remembered it the whole week. It was rough.

THERAPIST: Yes, but by not coming you don't achieve anything. You avoid the problem, but the problem doesn't disappear.

PATIENT: I know.

THERAPIST: So what was the problem that you were referring to?

PATIENT: Well, about my mother, how much I missed her. And then I remembered when I was young and I had a slumber party with my girlfriends. I was hoping that my father—you see, Dad woke up very early to go to work—wouldn't come into the room and get turned on by my sleeping girlfriends and do something. Of course I had that dream, that I told you about, when he raped me. . . .

THERAPIST: What are you trying to tell me? We have discussed all this before, this so-called rape dream, and all your sexual attractions—

PATIENT (interrupting): Yes, what I'm saying is that I was in love with my dad sexually. He treated me like a woman.

THERAPIST: Okay. Now, what about that?

PATIENT: Well, he threatened me. The dream was a threat of incest and I blame him for it.

THERAPIST: The dream was yours, not your father's.

PATIENT: Hm.

THERAPIST: You are putting the blame on your father. This is not going to solve your problem.

PATIENT: I have feelings. (giggling nervously)

THERAPIST (The therapist recapitulated in great detail what was discussed in the previous interview, and ended by saying): We clearly saw that emasculating men is in your hands. It is you who emasculates them. Today you seem to have shifted again. You tell me that your father threatens you, you place the emphasis on him rather than on yourself. You make him the villain who would be interested in your friends or in you. This is a projection and as such it won't help you understand your difficulties. Now, what we have here is that you either have wonderful relations with men or you emasculate them. We must try to figure out why you change.

PATIENT: Yeah . . . I'll try . . . (looking thoughtful) I love men. I

loved my father intensely, but I don't think of my father anymore. I love my mother very much. I don't write letters to my dad
anymore. I write only to Mom.

THERAPIST: What happened? Why this change?

PATIENT: This is a tendency in me. I love up to a point. I don't like
to be loved. After a while men become dependent, they want to
be married, so I get tired. I depart, I take a trip.

THERAPIST: Why do you run away? What are you afraid of?

PATIENT: I don't know. I get stifled.

THERAPIST: Who stifled you and kept you from being free?

PATIENT: I'm trying to think. . . . I feel sad. . . . I don't know. (crying)

THERAPIST: Come on . . . (The therapist offers her a box of tissues.)
. . . Don't run away from it all.

PATIENT: . . . I have this forsaken feeling again.

THERAPIST: Okay, let's hear about it.

PATIENT: I feel sorry for myself. I do want to blame my parents. I
don't want all this responsibility. . . . I felt stifled . . . that's
why I went to visit my sister (sighs). That was another trip I left
. . . (starts to cry again) . . . with.

THERAPIST: Go on.

PATIENT (crying): . . . Do you want to ask a question?

THERAPIST: Don't run away from these painful feelings. I know it's
hard for you, but blaming others won't help you.

PATIENT: I had guilt feelings about my mother. I fought with her all
the time . . . (crying) I was a bitch to my mother. . . . I ran to
Dad to punish my mother, and the thing is that I knew it at the
time. . . . I hurt my mother. I'd get in trouble on purpose, I
fought with my sister to get at my mother. I used all my weapons
to hurt her . . . I (sobbing), I always ruined the holidays for everybody. . . .

THERAPIST: I understand. Go on.

PATIENT: I did all sorts of bad things. I stole a lot when I was twelve.
. . . My father loved me, but my mother preferred my sister, and
later on I would have given everything to have my mother's affection. I never had it because I tried to alienate her, to hurt her.

THERAPIST: Yet you love your mother.

PATIENT (with much emphasis): Oh, I do love her!

THERAPIST: So why do you cry?

PATIENT: I feel guilty.

THERAPIST: As long as you know that you love her, that's all that counts.

PATIENT: But I don't know if she knows it.

THERAPIST: Well, let's not forget that you had your own reasons for doing what you did. You were in a predicament. You loved your father and you loved your mother, and you had to make a choice. That was very difficult. As soon as you loved your father, you started to find reasons why you disliked your mother and competed with her, but after a while you got caught because you loved your mother. How could a nice girl who loves her mother be so nasty to her? Of course you cry, of course you feel guilty. You are a sensitive person. Your problem is that you love people too much. You should be proud of that. Now, after a while you try to solve your dilemma. You become tired of the men, you emasculate the men, you take their genitals away from them, and you depart, you take a trip. The trouble is that all this does not solve your problem.

PATIENT: I see.

THERAPIST: Do you agree or not? Is what I said true? After all, you're the only one who knows.

PATIENT: Yes . . . but why do I keep on repeating all this? . . . (becoming teary again) I don't want to see my father go. . . .

THERAPIST: Why should this thought come to mind?

PATIENT: I think my dad is going to die. He's younger than my mother. He's only fifty-five. She's sixty.

THERAPIST: So why are you killing your father off?

PATIENT: I don't know. I have been thinking about my father's death for quite some time. He always dies first.

THERAPIST: Do you think of your mother's death?

PATIENT: No, my father always dies first, or if they die, they die together, but never my mother first.

THERAPIST: Now, what does your father die from in your fantasy?

PATIENT: Oh . . . of a massive heart attack, or in an automobile accident. It's very grotesque.

THERAPIST: Grotesque?

PATIENT: Yes, a gross thing. Grotesque . . . ugly.

THERAPIST: Yes, go on.

PATIENT: Car accident—

THERAPIST (*interrupting her*): But you say "grotesque." Why did you use the word "grotesque?"

PATIENT: Grotesque. (*giggling*)

THERAPIST: What is grotesque? Can you describe something which is grotesque? You giggle.

PATIENT: Well, a bloody bull fight . . . a physical handicap . . . a spastic who drools.

THERAPIST: So it has also to do with blood.

PATIENT: Oh, yes, blood. He's all crunched up. His body is all mangled, unrecognizable. That's what it is. . . .

THERAPIST: Anything else come to mind?

PATIENT (*hesitating*): . . . Well . . . my dad's genitals with the deep blue veins. Ugly . . . yeah . . . grotesque.

THERAPIST: Hm.

PATIENT: Yeah . . . but I don't think of my dad's genitals when I think of him in an automobile accident. I don't think of his genitals.

THERAPIST: Yes.

PATIENT: All of him is grotesque in my fantasy, not just his genitals.

THERAPIST: Twice you have emphasized that you do *not* think of his genitals in your fantasy.

PATIENT: Yes.

THERAPIST: Okay . . . maybe he doesn't have any genitals.

PATIENT (laughs): Oh, no!

THERAPIST: You seem to be amused.

PATIENT: I emasculated him once, so if—if I do a good job, he doesn't have any genitals. I do such a thorough job!

THERAPIST: Now what happens to them?

PATIENT: Well (*laughs*), I took them away.

THERAPIST: Yes.

PATIENT: Hm . . . he has none left.

THERAPIST: So you have them?

PATIENT: I . . . (*laughs*) I do. . . .

THERAPIST: Did you have such a fantasy?

PATIENT: . . . Now? . . . Well, I did think of how uncomfortable it would feel to have male genitals dangling between my legs.

THERAPIST: When did you have that fantasy?

PATIENT: Oh, fairly recently . . . with Tim. . . .

THERAPIST: You told me about it last time.

PATIENT: Did I tell you last time?

THERAPIST: You mean you forgot? When you said "my penis" of Tim's penis?

PATIENT: . . . Yes I said that. I remember now.

THERAPIST: Now, how did you get those genitals? You said you stole a lot when you were twelve.

PATIENT: I stole a lot (*laughs*). This is very complicated.

THERAPIST: No, it's very simple indeed.

PATIENT: Tell me.

THERAPIST: It's not up to me to explain it to you, but rather for you to figure it out from what you told me and what you remembered.

PATIENT: So I steal their genitals and I don't love them.

THERAPIST: Anymore?

PATIENT: I don't like to love.

THERAPIST: Not "don't like," but rather, "scared to love."

PATIENT: Well, it's that competition with my mother gives rise to these feelings of guilt, because I love my mother.

THERAPIST: So it's at such a time that the man becomes useless. You discard him—

PATIENT (*interrupting*): Yes, and I go away . . . and then I start all over again.

THERAPIST: Yes, the pattern is repeated.

PATIENT: I move.

THERAPIST: As you are moving again now.

PATIENT: Yes.

THERAPIST: Now, how are things with Mort?

PATIENT: Somewhat destructive. He just watches TV. He doesn't talk or communicate very much. I get angry. I do all his housekeeping. He doesn't appreciate it. I was mad at him all week. Well, we have our ups and downs. Some weeks are okay. This was a bad week. I said maybe we shouldn't see each other anymore. I'm a little wife but I don't want to marry him.

THERAPIST: Well, from what you say, maybe you shouldn't be putting all your eggs in one basket. Maybe you should have some other relationships.

PATIENT: You think so?

THERAPIST: If you don't want to marry him, and you think that you are not being appreciated, what's the point?

PATIENT: Well, maybe.

THERAPIST: Okay, it's time to stop now.

In this session the therapist does not let the patient get away with her projection of blaming her father, as he had let her do during the fourth interview. This being the eighth hour, he thought that the patient was ready to take full responsibility for her fantasies and her wishes. As expected, this produces a great deal of anxiety and tears, but, in addition, the patient produces a priceless fantasy about her father's death. The therapist exploits it by analyzing her use of the word "grotesque" and is able to clarify her need to emasculate men as a neurotic pattern.

The hour finally comes to an end with the discussion of her current relationship with Mort. At this point the therapist makes a mistake. Possibly because of his anxiety-provoking stance during the early part of the interview and all the tears which followed, the therapist becomes a bit too supportive and oversteps his neutral position by mentioning that, since her relationship with Mort seems so destructive, maybe she should have other relationships. This is for the patient to decide, not for the therapist to suggest. It is expected that he will pay a price for this mistake, and he does during the next interview.

NINTH INTERVIEW

The patient came to the interview looking agitated and depressed. She opened the ninth session by saying:

PATIENT: I pulled another boner. I broke off with Mort. He pays no attention to me. He views me as a piece of tail. It's foolish to be in a situation where he's interested in other women, like his ex-girlfriend, and uses me. I broke up with him, yet I feel bad. You said that the relationship with him was destructive and that I could date other men. I thought of what we talked about, my mother and all that. Tony also said that I was a good piece of ass. I want more from life than just to sleep around with men.(*starting to cry*)

THERAPIST: I'm intrigued seeing you cry. Why are you crying?

PATIENT: I cried all day. I was afraid that you would make a big deal out of my ending my relationship with Mort. I want to decide what to do with my own life. I don't want you to think that you affect my life.

The therapist at this point emphasized that he thought her tears had to do with two entirely different features. The first one had to do with him. She wanted him to feel sorry for her. This was her old position of becoming the victim. The second aspect had to do with the sad feelings that were aroused as a result of her breaking up with Mort. The therapist also emphasized that it was up to her to decide what she wanted to do with her life, and that he in no way felt that she should or should not see other men.

After a while the patient seemed to calm down, so the therapist thought it appropriate to return to the subject of her feelings for her mother that had been discussed during the previous session. He went on as follows:

THERAPIST: Let's go back to what we were discussing last week, about your mother.

PATIENT: Okay. Yes . . . you mean about my feeling embarrassed to look at my mother after I had heard them having intercourse during the night?

THERAPIST (*This was not what the therapist had in mind, but he was interested in the patient's associations, so he went on*): All right, what about that?

PATIENT: . . . I don't know.

THERAPIST: What comes to mind?

PATIENT: I was angry at them for making so much noise. I was angry at both of them, but I felt only embarrassed about my mother.

THERAPIST: Now this is interesting. Why embarrassed only about your mother. What does the word "embarrassed" mean in this context?

PATIENT: . . . Well (*laughing*), a comparison comes to mind. When one is on stage and makes a complete fool of herself. I'm embarrassed for such a person! (*laughing*)

THERAPIST: So your mother made a fool of herself.

PATIENT: Hm.

THERAPIST: What aspect of your mother's behavior did you feel embarrassed about?

PATIENT: Oh . . . the way she expressed herself during intercourse. She sounded as if she was in pain, instead of expressing pleasure. . . . I . . . I figured that she was uncoordinated.

THERAPIST: There we are again! You say these things by using headlines. We have talked about this tendency in you. What exactly do you mean by the word "uncoordinated?"

PATIENT (*giggling*): Well . . . I didn't think that my mother was very good in bed. (*giggling continues*)

THERAPIST: What was so embarrassing and so funny? You giggle.

PATIENT: . . . Maybe . . . maybe that I heard her, that I overheard what was going on.

THERAPIST: What are you thinking about right now? Don't try to run away.

PATIENT: . . . I'm trying to think why I was embarrassed.

THERAPIST: Don't try so hard. Be spontaneous. Now we have "embarrassment," "in pain," "uncoordination."

PATIENT: I wanted to talk to her, to tell her. . . .

THERAPIST: Did you tell her?

PATIENT: No . . . maybe having intercourse. . . .

THERAPIST: Yes, go on.

PATIENT: Having intercourse with my dad. Maybe she did it to hurt me.

THERAPIST: To hurt you? Hm! It was she who was in pain. But let's pursue this point of her trying to hurt you.

At this point the patient appeared to be very anxious. She tried repeatedly to run away from the subject but the therapist wouldn't let her do it because he was sure she was avoiding some important and anxiety-provoking fantasies.

THERAPIST: You mentioned the dream, your dream about having intercourse with your father. We also know that you had seen your father's genitals. Did you compare yourself with your mother?

PATIENT: . . . I think so. (*blushing*)

THERAPIST: When you become intellectual, you are running away, yet you blush. I don't expect you to give me some kind of a definite answer.

PATIENT: . . . Like . . . I try to please men, like my dad. Maybe I tried to convince my dad that I was better than my mother. She was always asleep. . . . I felt embarrassed for her, yet I was a virgin then. I was like my mother.

THERAPIST: What do you mean by that? Do you mean that you were both uncoordinated?

PATIENT (*emphatically*): Oh, no! I'm not.

THERAPIST: You are coordinated, and your mother is not. So you are—

PATIENT (*interrupting*): Better!

THERAPIST: Ah! Better!

PATIENT: Hm . . . hm. . . .

THERAPIST: Now, what do you mean by "better"? In what way are you better?

PATIENT: Well.

THERAPIST: Yeah?

PATIENT: . . . I know things. I knew how to make my dad happy—cooking, talking to him, his drink.

THERAPIST: True, but these things are not connected with sexual intercourse, which is what we are talking about now.

PATIENT: Right.

THERAPIST: Better in what way?

PATIENT: Better in bed. (*laughing*)

THERAPIST: Yes.

PATIENT: Now I know I'm good in bed, but then I didn't know much about sex.

THERAPIST: It's the thought that counts, not what really happened.

PATIENT: Okay.

THERAPIST: In what way are you *now* good in bed?

PATIENT (*blushing*): . . . You want me to explain?

THERAPIST: I mean, in terms of being different from and better than your mother.

PATIENT: Well, I'm not in pain. I express my pleasure. I'm more affectionate, more loving. I'm much more coordinated.

THERAPIST: So every time you are "affectionate," "loving," "not in pain," "expressing pleasure," "coordinated," and "good in bed," the thought comes to your mind that you are *better* than your mother, that you are beating your mother in the sexual game.

PATIENT: Yes, I do. (*emphatically*)

THERAPIST: But now, what ultimately happens every time you are good in bed, every time you win?

PATIENT: What do you mean?

THERAPIST: I mean precisely that—

PATIENT (*interrupting*): Oh, I see. I leave.

THERAPIST: Indeed, you leave! Actually, two things happen. You leave, and I quote you now, "you become disgusted by the man's genitals, you take them away, you emasculate the men." Now, you do all this because you can't live happily with the notion of your victory over your mother. You feel guilty.

PATIENT: . . . Yeah! In reality it takes a year or so. This victory takes a long time.

THERAPIST: Yes, it takes time, but it eventually catches up with you. At first you are loving, good in bed, coordinated, and enjoy it all. But soon, as time goes by, these other feelings creep up. After all, isn't that what happened with Tim? Didn't you become turned off and leave him?

PATIENT: Yes.

THERAPIST: Yes, and after you became pregnant and had good sex with Jim, you threw him out and you rushed back home to have your abortion. You rushed back *home*. Now the question is, why do you do that? Why is it so important? Why the urge? You didn't have to go home for that.

PATIENT: That's true. . . . I don't know why.

THERAPIST: Every time you are victorious, every time you beat your mother, what happens?

PATIENT: I move.

THERAPIST: Yes. You move to get away from the men whom you emasculate. If you win, what happens to the other person, to the loser?

PATIENT: I emasculate the man.

THERAPIST: No, that is not the point. Yes, you do emasculate the man, but the battle is with your mother. It is she who is the loser. Two people battle, one wins. What happens to the loser?

PATIENT: I leave.

THERAPIST: So the other person is not there for you anymore.

PATIENT: She's not there. . . .

THERAPIST: What does it mean if she's not there?

PATIENT: I won. I'm the winner. She's the loser. (*grimacing*)

THERAPIST: She's not there anymore. . . .

PATIENT: I don't want to see it . . . it hurts.

THERAPIST: Of course, because it *is* painful.

PATIENT: I write to my mother, not to my father.

THERAPIST: Of course! Exactly. (*encouraging her to go on*)

PATIENT: I don't want to think about it. I don't want to see it. I can't.

THERAPIST: It *is* very difficult.

PATIENT: I can't. I won't! (*laughs nervously*)

THERAPIST: It is important to look at it. Not because I say so, but because it is the truth.

PATIENT: Okay. I wipe her out when I win. . . .

THERAPIST: When you win, you wipe the other person out. You do this with both men and women. If you wipe the other person out, and that includes your mother, then the other person doesn't exist anymore.

PATIENT: I keep on repeating it.

THERAPIST: Yes, because there is a part of you that does not want to wipe her out. If she disappears, she dies!

PATIENT: Sure! Oh, God, this is hard!

THERAPIST: Yes. . . .

PATIENT: But she's still there. She hasn't died.

THERAPIST: How do you know that she's still there?

PATIENT: Well, she is.

THERAPIST: In reality yes, but how do you know?

PATIENT: I repeat the pattern.

THERAPIST: Yes, but you don't know. If you wiped her out, maybe she *is* dead. Isn't it then time to go home to see if she's still around? To reassure yourself that you haven't wiped her out, that she's not really dead? And this frightens you. Okay, let's not forget that all this is in your mind. I know that is difficult. Now, by wiping your mother out, you are left with the thought that you don't have a mother anymore.

PATIENT: But I'll be free then!

THERAPIST: Come now! How can you be free when we know that you love your mother, that you write only to her, that you are sad in the airport when she doesn't give you a second kiss? You know that if you lost your mother you'd be very sad. Isn't it true?

PATIENT: If my mother were dead, oh, God! . . . (*teary*)

THERAPIST: There you are! Now, that is why you have to go home—
to make sure, double sure, that you have not wiped out your
mother, the mother whom you love and who is so important to
you.

PATIENT: Yes. Even if I win the battle, I go home because I love her
so much. So I go home to make sure that she's around! This is
why I go.

THERAPIST: Precisely, over and over. Now, none of this is real. It is
all inside your head. You did *not* sleep with your father. You do
not know that you are better than your mother. You did *not* really
beat your mother. This is all a neurotic pattern that gets activated
slowly every time you are successful with men, every time you
compare yourself to your mother, every time you have the
thought that you wipe her out. What would a little girl do without her mommy whom she loves?

PATIENT (*teary*): Yes.

THERAPIST: Yes, that mother who is so important to you that you are
in tears at the thought of losing her, as you are in tears right now.
This is why you stop your relationships with all these men.

PATIENT (*crying*): Yes, I know. How do I stop all this?

THERAPIST: By doing the hard work that we have been doing today.
Do some thinking about it next week, and don't forget that all
this is only in your mind. Now I shall have to be away for
about four weeks.

PATIENT: Okay.

This interview shows clearly several aspects of STAPP technique which have already been encountered before, but which all
come nicely together during this session. These include (1) the return to the focus by the therapist ("Let us go back to what we were
discussing," etc.); (2) challenging the patient's globalizing and
headlining defenses by insisting on the specific meaning, fantasies,
and details of certain key words which are used by the patient, such
as "embarrassing" and "uncoordinated"; (3) clarifying the focal
conflict with her mother, and the thought of defeating her mother
in sexual matters; (4) the persistence in surveying the material and,
despite the patient's efforts to run away, keeping her squarely on
the focal conflict; and (5) insisting on tying all the material together
and pointing to the desire to defeat her mother with the threat of

losing her, and clarifying the pattern of her behavior in reference to men as well as her mother.

Finally, and only after everything appears to look clear and the patient bursts into tears at the realization of what she is doing, the therapist is supportive, emphasizing that she is working hard and that all these thoughts constitute a neurotic pattern which, after all, is only inside the patient's head and has nothing to do with reality. It is clear that the interview ends on a very positive note.

At this point the therapist should speculate on what to expect for the following hour. Usually after such a difficult interview, when everything seems to have fallen into place, there must be some sort of dramatic relief from all this tension. This is precisely what happened in the tenth session.

TENTH INTERVIEW

The patient, looking quite relieved, announced that Mort had called her and asked her out for a drink. He begged her to resume their relationship. She laid down her conditions, and he seemed to have accepted them all. She also talked about having made arrangements to get a new job with more pay, and about planning to buy a new car. She said that, generally speaking, she was feeling very much better.

The therapist acknowledged that he also felt that considerable progress had been made and asked her how much she thought their joint work might be responsible for all these changes. He also asked her to tell what she had learned about herself.

She said that she knew that she loved her mother and that she understood the pattern about competition and the need to go home. Although somewhat unclear about the pattern of emasculating men, she felt that she did not have the urge to be attracted to "sick" men anymore, and that her relationship with Mort, although not ideal, was now much more on a give-and-take basis. She was very pleased with herself and emphasized that she felt proud to be a woman, and realized that all these problems did not upset her as much, since she understands what she does and why she does it. It appeared to the therapist that indeed her problems were on the verge of being solved. The session ended on a very positive note.

ELEVENTH INTERVIEW

The patient looked relaxed and happy. She smiled at her therapist and said:

PATIENT: I feel great. I really feel fine. I've been thinking that I'll be a success in my life. It feels good to go over things. I've learned a great deal from what we discussed here. The only problems that remain are realistic ones like my job, moving, and so on. I did go out, by the way, with another guy.
THERAPIST: I see!
PATIENT: I don't like him very much. He's kind of a creep, but I did go out for a beer and a drink.

She continued to discuss her date in some detail, and to emphasize that, although she was not planning to marry Mort, she enjoyed their new relationship. Then she added:

PATIENT: I feel I'll start to blame you for something.
THERAPIST: Oh? We must hear about that.

The therapist nevertheless thought that he should first clarify his position in reference to her going out with other men, and emphasized that it was up to her to decide how and with whom she should go out now that she knew what her feelings were all about. He kept in mind, however, her statement about blaming him and planned to come back to it later on in this interview. After some additional discussion, the patient went on as follows:

PATIENT: As to my therapy, I think a great deal about it, and when I do, the first thing that comes to my mind is this emasculation business. It is the most upsetting thing that I've discovered about myself so far. This issue about my mother is also very difficult, but I can deal with it. But this emasculation stuff . . . I want to understand it completely before we quit, before we stop psychotherapy.
THERAPIST: This is a good point, but we are not stopping today.
PATIENT: Yes, I know.
THERAPIST: Let's start thinking about it.

PATIENT: I know we won't continue psychotherapy for another year.

THERAPIST: We don't need to.

PATIENT: Yes, I know that, but I do want to have enough to think about before you go away. Yet I look forward to this break. I don't want you to go, but also I do, because I'm not as dependent on you as my roommate is on her psychiatrist. Well, anyway, I had a dream. I was feeling so good about myself. Yet I had a bad dream—which brought to mind all the unpleasant things. It was about my supervisor. You know, she's a real puritan virgin. She knows all about my follies, my escapades, and she doesn't agree with me. I don't expect her to. She's a sick girl.

THERAPIST: Now what was the dream about?

PATIENT: Jane, that's my supervisor's name, and I had gone out drinking and then we went to a party at some of her friends. I soon remembered that I had to go back to my place to feed my dog, but all these people at the party turned out to be against me. They were all very hostile. One woman called me a "slut," another called me "dumb." It was as if Jane had told all these people about my life, about my sleeping around. At the end I remember begging a man to give me a lift and he wouldn't give me the time of day. Everyone, both men and women, glared at me and said all these mean things. I woke up in an awful sweat . . . yech! And here I was feeling so good about myself last week, and I'm having such a crummy and destructive dream.

THERAPIST: Now, I'm not at all sure that it's as destructive as you think. What was the most striking feature about the dream?

PATIENT: The most important? Well, it was that all these people were against me and Jane had made them turn against me. You see, Jane and I disagree on many issues. We have different life-styles and all that.

THERAPIST: It was a woman who made people turn against you.

PATIENT: Right.

THERAPIST: And this frightened you.

PATIENT: Yes.

THERAPIST: So we have a powerful woman who can create a lot of unpleasantness for you. Does this remind you of anything?

PATIENT: . . . As we discussed already, competition, the triangle between two women and a man. If I feel like that about my mother and I go about emasculating men—

THERAPIST (*interrupting*): Just a minute! Not so fast! Let's stick to the dream, okay? You describe Jane as being "puritanical," "sick," "disapproving of you," and "powerful." What is it that she knows about you and how did she find out?

PATIENT: In the dream?

THERAPIST: No, in reality.

PATIENT: Oh, I tell her.

THERAPIST: The question is, why do you tell her?

PATIENT: I tell everybody.

THERAPIST: The question is, why do you tell everybody, and her in particular? (*laughter*)

PATIENT: Well, that's a problem.

THERAPIST: I don't say that it's a problem. I'm just asking you.

PATIENT: Okay . . . well, we discuss all these things and she says (*patient imitating Jane's voice*), "Oh, I'll never sleep with a man," and I say, "Oh, I've been sleeping with a lot of guys and I like it. I enjoy sex. I can't see why you're afraid of it." I even told her that I sleep with Mort, and that I'm on birth control pills . . . .

THERAPIST: What does Jane look like?

PATIENT: She's a lovely girl. Attractive, tall, thin, twenty-five, smart.

THERAPIST: Competitive?

PATIENT: Oh, yeah! Very competitive.

THERAPIST: If the two of you were to compete, as you do, who wins?

PATIENT: As far as I'm concerned . . . you mean if we competed over a man? I definitely think (*smiling*) that she would win. Definitely!

THERAPIST: I am not so sure about that, looking at the expression on your face.

PATIENT (*continuing to smile*): Now, if one of our male supervisors or, you know, one of our superiors were interested in us, someone that I'd like to date, let's say, then she wins because she has the status. She's also my superior and she's better educated. She has an MA. I'm not as smart as she is. I don't have the status, I have no MA. Oh, I don't think that she's more attractive, but she has the status, that I know. My personality is nice. Basically (*laughing*), basically I'm a more squared-away individual and I'm sure I'd be a much better and happier dating partner, but on that status stuff (*laughing*) . . . .

THERAPIST (*also laughing*): Wait a minute! If a man, one of your superiors, let's say, wanted to go out with a girl who has status, Jane wins. But if he was going out with a girl who has a good personality and was a good *sexual* partner, you win.

PATIENT: True! (*smiling*) . . . not just sexual. I mean—

THERAPIST (*interrupting*): I know. *I* emphasized the word "sexual." You talked about being well adjusted, good personality, and so on, but it was *you* who kept on talking about sex with Jane, as a result of which a difference of opinion emerged between the two of you. Isn't that so?

PATIENT: Yes.

THERAPIST: In the area of sex, therefore, there is a battle between the two of you. She is puritanical, you're not. You kept using the word "sex" with Jane. You told her about your birth control pills, sleeping with Mort, enjoying intercourse. Why did you do that?

PATIENT: I don't know.

THERAPIST: Come now, of course you do. In the area of personality there might be differences of opinion, as far as who is smarter there might be conflicting notions, but in the area of sex—

PATIENT: I'm better! (*smiling*)

THERAPIST: Of course, in the area of sex you beat Jane every time.

PATIENT: Yes (*laughing*), I do.

THERAPIST: So *you* used sex to hit Jane over the head.

PATIENT: Oh, yes, and I hit her quite often, again and again. (*general laughter*)

THERAPIST: . . . Okay, now that is aggressive.

PATIENT: I pulled another boner. The other day she said, "Oh, I'm so constipated." She's very neurotic, you know, so I said to her, "Why don't you go to see a psychiatrist?"

THERAPIST: I see! Hm!

PATIENT: I said to her, "Oh, I hope I'm not offending you." I'll apologize to her for saying that, because I feel embarrassed about it.

THERAPIST: You mean to say that it is offensive to see a psychiatrist?

PATIENT: For Jane it is. Yes, it is!

THERAPIST: Just a minute. This is also a way of hitting me over the head, isn't it?

PATIENT: Why? (*surprised*)

THERAPIST: If it is an insult to see a psychiatrist which will upset Jane, and you have to apologize for it, and since I am a psychiatrist, then aren't you also trying to hit me over the head, and don't we know the reason why?

PATIENT: Yes, because you're going away. (*laughing*)

THERAPIST: Kill two birds with one stone! Send Jane to me! (*laughing*) . . . Okay, now let's get back to this important dream of yours, and your questions about it. What we know up to now is that you use sex aggressively because you know that in that area, you win.

PATIENT: Yes, this is the only area I win in.

THERAPIST: And then you have the dream. Now, what does the dream tell us?

PATIENT: Jane destroyed me. My weapon against her is also destroyed because all the men are against me.

THERAPIST: Precisely.

PATIENT: Jane is a big thorn in my side.

THERAPIST: Now, let's go back to your question earlier in the hour.

PATIENT: You mean about emasculation?

THERAPIST: Yes . . . you have answered it, you know!

PATIENT: Well, Jane made all the men turn against me.

THERAPIST: In the dream, yes. But in reality it is you who are against the men, you throw them away.

PATIENT: Not all the time.

THERAPIST: No, only at the time when you feel forced to emasculate the man. Now, I think that we know the reason why you do.

PATIENT: Because I win.

THERAPIST: Of course, because you win! Now, when you do, the other woman, Jane in this case, becomes angry and what does she do to you? She uses her power to destroy your weapon, and makes the men turn against you. Like a magical witch, she makes the whole world turn hostile and you are scared of her. This fear wakes you up and you discover that you are in an "awful sweat."

PATIENT: Yes.

THERAPIST: Now, let's see. If this powerful woman threatens you and accuses you because she wants to retaliate for your victory, don't you have a wonderful alibi?

PATIENT: . . . Oh, oh. He turns me off! (*laughing*)

THERAPIST (*laughing*): Not only he turns you off, but just look at him, Jane. He doesn't have anything down there. He is emasculated.

PATIENT: Yeah. (*continuing to laugh*)

THERAPIST: I suspect you used this alibi way back when you were little. Who were you so frightened of when you were young?

PATIENT: My mother.

THERAPIST: Yes, as we have already discovered. Now, was your mother ever in reality as angry at you as Jane was in the dream?

PATIENT: . . . No, not really. Well, we really competed. Once she said that she got along with her mother as badly as we did. I felt terrible. I felt like a heel. I cried and cried.

THERAPIST: We know why you cried, and why you felt guilty. Because you competed with her and because by comparing yourself wih her, and by deciding that you were better than she was in bed, you started to feel scared that she would retaliate. So immediately you started thinking of your alibi. Mainly that the man was emasculated and no sex was possible. What strikes me, however, is that your mother was mild, not as you portrayed Jane to be in your dream.

PATIENT: Well, yes, she was mild.

THERAPIST: I suspect that you exaggerated Jane's nastiness in the dream because you had a mild mother. If you had a mother who was an ogre it would have been an even battle, but because your mother was mild you had to exaggerate your guilt feelings and fear of punishment.

PATIENT: But I don't let her beat me.

THERAPIST: You don't, but you take another roundabout way. You create your own punishment to stop you from the temptations of having sex with men, like your father, and of defeating your mother by being better than she is in bed. Then you emasculate the men and say to your mother, "Look, mother, what sex? There was no sex with this kind of a man—my dad. I'm innocent. No sex with him—he's emasculated."

PATIENT: Yes, emasculation always follows the dream.

THERAPIST: Yes, the dream of your father, the dream of the two faceless men, and so on. It's all there!

PATIENT (smiling): Hm.

THERAPIST: So, you see, we have learned a great deal from this most interesting dream of yours!

PATIENT: I begin to know my weapons now that I understand what I do. It all seems to be okay.

THERAPIST: Very good! So I'll see you in four weeks.

PATIENT: Have a good time.

THERAPIST: Thank you.

It is of interest that the analysis of this dream gives the partici- pants a wonderful opportunity to work out all the details of the psychodynamic problem which seems to have been completely re- solved. What remains to be done now is to see how the patient is going to react during the therapist's absence. If all goes well, the therapy can be terminated.

This is indeed what happened. Except for some minor prob- lems with Mort, the patient did very well during the month's sepa- ration. As a result of this, it was decided that the treatment should end after two more sessions.

During the twelfth hour several issues, such as the emascu- lation of men, competition with women, relations with other women, and problems at work, were all discussed in some detail.

The last interview was typical of a STAPP patient. It was essen- tially future-oriented. She talked about her plans, and although she expressed some sadness at the prospect of not seeing her therapist anymore, she said that she was ready to stop. During the last few minutes she enumerated her achievements and ended by saying that she wanted to be a "good wife and mother."

Nine months after the end of the treatment she wrote a letter to the therapist, saying that she was planning to move in six months' time. She wrote that she was eager to verbalize to him all the won- derful feelings that she had experienced after the end of her treat- ment. She emphasized that she felt very good about herself. She enjoyed her work much more than before and felt that she was good at it. Her main emphasis, however, was on all the things which she had learned about herself—which she recapitulated.

FOLLOW-UP INTERVIEW

Thirteen months after termination the therapist had a follow-up interview with the patient. Her appearance had changed in a strik- ing manner. She was much more poised, very fashionably dressed, and looked very relaxed and happy. She opened the interview by saying:

PATIENT: I feel very positive. I haven't emasculated Mort. We have been living together and have a very satisfactory sexual relationship. He gives much more to me than he used to, and I know that it will be very hard to leave him, but I am determined to go. I have an excellent new job opportunity and I know I could never marry Mort. I want to meet and marry someone who is better educated than I am, who can teach me new things. Mort is quite limited, but he's a nice person.

THERAPIST: Now, in reference to your therapy, what do you remember about it?

PATIENT: I feel very proud of myself and of what I accomplished. When I have a problem, I talk to myself and I figure things out all by myself. I've changed so much. My relations with people have improved greatly. I can see how the therapy worked.

Five years later, in response to a questionnaire which was sent to the patient to assess her progress, she sent a letter, some excerpts of which are included here. She wrote:

"I'm still single. I want a man to settle down with. I'm much more sure of the kind of man I want. I know that you are interested in my present attitude toward men, but honestly, I don't think that I have a problem any longer.

"I have been working. I am confident and effective. . . . I am a very capable woman. It's hard to explain succinctly how great a life it is, and how much I have changed since I was in treatment with you . . . .

"Sometimes I feel low, but other times life is great. My parents are alive and well. I really enjoyed those six months and I really liked you, and I wish to call you by your first name. Thanks a lot. I wish I could talk to you in person."

In terms of her answers to our follow-up questionnaire, here is a sample:

Why did you seek treatment?
Insecurity. Difficulty with men. The sicker the man, the more appealing. I didn't like myself. I had an abortion.
How do you feel now?
At times very good. At times slightly depressed. Hopeful of a good future.
Self-esteem?
Self-esteem is very high. At times I feel lonely, but I am a much better person, capable, strong.

New relations? and work relations?

Have many good women friends. I am a good responsible worker.

Interpersonal difficulties?

None.

Learning during therapy

My mother was a big problem as a result of a triangle.

Problem solving?

Understanding my relations with men.

Recent changes

Life is good, mood is pretty good almost constantly. I don't have attractions for sick men anymore.

In sum, one would say that the patient's psychological problems seem to have been resolved and that she is leading a happy and meaningful life. This is a source of great satisfaction to her therapist.

Appendix II

The previous case example depicted the process of STAPP with a female patient. To balance things out I shall now present the treatment of a male patient, not only to demonstrate the unfolding of this kind of treatment between two participants of the same sex but also because this patient was thought to be more severely incapacitated than some of the individuals who have been already described in this book. For the readers who are interested in DSM-III diagnostic criteria, this patient would fall into the "obsessive personality disorder" category.

EVALUATION INTERVIEW

A 26-year-old business school student came to the psychiatric clinic complaining of incapacitating procrastination, inability to prepare himself for his examinations, and failure to submit papers on time. As a result of these problems he was afraid that he would be dismissed from the school, or that he would be at least placed on probation. These difficulties had become progressively worse as the time of his examinations approached, and the situation gave rise to intense anxiety and depressive feelings. He was afraid that he would never be able to get an MBA degree, yet he felt completely paralyzed, confused, and unable to do anything about this situation. Similar difficulties, but in a much milder form, had existed before he got his BA degree. He went on as follows:

PATIENT: There is something peculiar about all this. You see, objectively there is no reality to it. My grades are excellent. I graduated with honors from college and my teachers tell me that I am doing fine, but I suspect that they really do not understand how little I know. The only thing which annoys them is my inability to submit my papers on time. I must tell you that I received behavior modification treatment for these problems for several months, but it did me no good at all, and I stopped it. I come here now for help. It is my last resort.

The patient was the oldest of three children. He had a brother four years younger and a sister five years younger than himself. He came from a closely knit, well-to-do family. He was born in Italy and was in the United States for his education. His parents lived in Rome. His father was 57 years old, a successful engineer, but he was dissatisfied with his profession because he always wanted to be a "businessman." Although he was described as being rigid in his dealings with the other members of his family, the father was very lenient with the patient, whom he considered to be extremely intelligent, capable of succeeding in anything he attempted to do. This attitude was in direct contrast with his feelings for his younger son, whom he viewed as being lazy, good-for-nothing, and destined to fail in life, and whom, for all intents and purposes, he ignored.

The mother, to whom the patient was very attached, was very attentive and loving to all of her children. When the evaluator asked the patient to describe his mother, he said that she was "beautiful," "sentimental," "fresh," and very "coquettish." He added also that his mother was quite disturbed by the existing rift between her younger son and his father and tried to act as an "in-between."

He was very fond of his younger sister. Tall and thin, she was very much like his girlfriend, Susan, who was attending college in Chicago and to whom he was thinking of becoming engaged.

Although he emphasized that he did not remember many episodes from his childhood in Italy, he said that in general he was happy. He was an excellent student in grade school and had a close friend for whom he would make all sorts of sacrifices because he greatly valued his friendship, and he would always visit him first whenever he returned to Italy, even before going to see his parents.

During the interview the patient seemed to be somewhat tense, tended to go into many details as he described his symptoms, but interacted well with the evaluator despite this uneasiness, speaking spontaneously, and gesturing extensively to emphasize the points that he was making. He was clearly aware that his problems were psychological and was motivated to change so that he could, as he put it, "once and for all free myself from this paralyzing difficulty which threatens to ruin my future career." As the evaluation interview went on, the following exchange took place:

EVALUATOR: You said that you did not remember many episodes from your childhood, yet you emphasize that you felt happy. Why is it?

PATIENT: Yes, I did. I don't know why.

EVALUATOR: For example, you mentioned that you were four years older than your brother. Do you remember his birth?

PATIENT: Yes, I do. I remember that my mother was gone and I was very unhappy. My father took me to the hospital and I saw my brother. He looked like a chimpanzee. I have always felt pity for him.

EVALUATOR: So, you do remember some episodes from the past. Do you remember the birth of your sister?

PATIENT: No, but I recall going to her room. She looked like a beautiful doll.

EVALUATOR: From what you said you had different but essentially good relationships with your parents.

PATIENT: In contrast to my brother, yes, I did.

EVALUATOR: Well, you seemed to have been your father's favorite.

PATIENT: (*interrupting*): I was the favorite of both my parents and my grandparents also. You see, I was the oldest; they did also love my sister very much.

EVALUATOR: Who was your favorite parent?

PATIENT: . . . (*He was silent for several minutes.*)

EVALUATOR: Is this such a difficult question?

PATIENT: It definitely is.

EVALUATOR: Well, you may not have to answer it today, but I can assure you that you will have to answer it during your psychotherapy.

PATIENT: (*sighing*): I see.

EVALUATOR: You sigh—is this a sigh of relief?

PATIENT: It is a difficult decision because I have such a different relationship with both of my parents. With my father there is his attitude that I can do anything I want, which I like but which frustrates me when I have the academic difficulties which I have already talked about. With my mother it is different. She deals with me as if I were a grown-up. She confides in me. I am flattered but I also feel uneasy. My father has my success in mind.

EVALUATOR: So, having difficulties academically interferes with your father's expectations of your success. Is success then the issue, or putting it in a different way, do you want to fail so as to escape from this attitude of your father's? Liberate yourself from it? Does this issue ring any bells for you?

PATIENT: It rings too many bells.

EVALUATOR: Let's hear about one or two!

PATIENT: It reminds me of an experience that I had as a teenager. I was a good chess player. Well—the reality was I was an excellent chess player. I used to play simultaneously with twenty people—you know, moving from one chessboard to another—and I would win. When my father heard about it and started to suggest that I should join the Italian chess club and compete internationally, I gave up chess, and I never touched it again.

EVALUATOR: This is a very good example of what I had in mind.

The evaluation interview continued with a systematic history taking, the highlights of which have already been described.

In the evaluator's mind it was clear that the patient fulfilled the criteria for STAPP and also that the focus of the treatment had to be the unresolved conflictual Oedipal feelings of the patient for his parents, with success or failure, academically and otherwise, being the results of these conflicts. He proceeded to present his ideas to the patient in order to obtain his agreement.

EVALUATOR: I think that the symptoms of anxiety and depression which result from your procrastination and fear of academic failure, and which bring you to the clinic, seem to be related to the feelings which you have about your parents in this "success–failure" issue. Realistically, you are doing well academically. I propose, therefore, that we make the focus of your therapy your emotional conflicts with your parents and concentrate on their resolution. If, as a result of the therapy, your academic difficulties can also be eliminated, so much the better. In any case, I hope

that you will be able to get much insight into these family relations which have created many problems for you over the years.
Are you willing to agree with this formulation of mine, to examine
these issues over a short period of time?

PATIENT: Yes! Yes, I do. I really didn't expect any immediate change
in my problems at the business school. I agree with you and I am
eager to get to work. You say "over a short period of time." What
do you mean? How long?

EVALUATOR: I am glad to hear what you say. Let us make plans to
start as soon as you have seen another evaluator. This is part of
our research about this short-term psychotherapy. As far as its
length is concerned, I cannot answer your question precisely because I do not know how long it would take for you and your
therapist to work these problems through. I would suppose it would
take a few months time on a once-a-week basis. Is that all right?

PATIENT: Yes. That's fine.

The patient was seen by a female psychiatrist as a part of the
research design of STAPP evaluation to assess the criteria for selection and the therapeutic focus as well as to specify outcome criteria.
The second evaluator agreed that he was a good candidate for STAPP
and the focus should be the unresolved Oedipal problem. She specified the following criteria for successful outcome: (1) improvement
in his procrastination and in his anxiety and depression symptoms,
(2) ability to perform academic work as exemplified by his obtaining
his MBA degree, (3) insight into his relations with his father and
freedom from the success–failure dilemma, (4) insight into his relationships with his mother, and (5) establishment of a meaningful
relationship with his current girlfriend or with another woman.

In addition, the patient was asked if he would agree to have his
therapy videotaped. This he accepted to do, and he eagerly signed
an "informal consent form."

FIRST INTERVIEW

PATIENT: I felt uneasy and anxious about meeting you and talking
with you. It was much easier to talk with the other lady, whose
name I don't know. I saw her last week.

THERAPIST: She was Dr. K. Did this difficulty with me have to do with my being a man? Do you have an easier time with women?

PATIENT: No, no. In school I get along well with my male teachers, except with those who think that I am so great and who do not understand my difficulties and my shortcomings. As I told you, I had behavior therapy which did me no good, but I liked my therapist. He was also a male.

THERAPIST: Do you feel, then, that I did not understand your problem and that made you feel uneasy?

PATIENT: In some way, yes, because you want to focus the treatment in a different area. You also minimize my academic fears.

THERAPIST: So you view me like your father and those professors of yours who don't understand your fears.

PATIENT: In a way. Yes.

THERAPIST: Yet your uneasiness may also signify an anxiety about looking into, and resolving, the problems with your parents. In any case, I am not your father. I am not your professor. I am here to help you understand yourself.

The therapist has just, at the outset of the therapy, been able to make a parent-transference link, which as has already been discussed, is a crucial technical aspect of short-term dynamic psychotherapy.

THERAPIST: (continuing): You did mention having behavior therapy before. Can you give me some more details about it?

PATIENT: As you know, I have been very anxious about writing papers and preparing myself for quizzes and exams. I was confused, almost paralyzed one time when I was late in submitting a paper. One of my teachers, Dr. W, called me in his office and said, "You are one of our best students. Why do you undermine your work by not writing your paper? Write anything you want. Just one page long will suffice and I'll give you a good grade." Well, you know, I could not write a single line. I stayed up all night, I was exhausted, and I wrote three lines in all. I said to myself, "The mountain that roared and produced a mouse." I thought of getting a leave of absence but my professors were against it. They think that I know so much more than I think I do. They think that I am terrific. (He looked very sad as he was talking.)

THERAPIST: So, they all behave like your father.

PATIENT: . . . Hm. . . . Yes, they are *so* understanding. One of them used the exact words of my father's: "You can do anything that you want if you put your mind into it." I felt very irritable inside. I thought, "How do you know?" I am expected to produce. One of my teachers said "Write anything; write crap." I felt insulted. Imagine that *I* should write crap!

THERAPIST: Do you view your father as being insulting when he praises you?

PATIENT: No, but I always thought that he had untenably high standards and wanted me to have the same. I become self-critical, but I know that if I did not have my father's prodding I wouldn't have been able to get anywhere. I'd be lost. I'd be a failure.

THERAPIST: If you didn't have it you will be free, and you will become like your brother. You will be ignored by your father, free to do what you like.

PATIENT: (*smiling, and ignoring the analogy with his brother*): I had to keep up with his high standards. Sometimes I would feel so self-conscious, particularly when my mother praised me. I would feel ridiculous.

THERAPIST: Ridiculous?

PATIENT: You see, my mother was a good dancer, and once when she saw me dancing she said that I was "moving very well." It was around the age of thirteen or so. But I remember that as soon as she started complimenting me I wouldn't want to dance. I stopped altogether a few weeks later. I have never danced since. Susan, my girlfriend, is upset with me about it, but I cannot. I will not.

THERAPIST: Like not playing chess.

PATIENT: Yes.

THERAPIST: Can we hear more about all this?

PATIENT: I don't remember my childhood. I told you that already. (*irritably*)

THERAPIST: It is surprising that you wouldn't remember something ·which happened at the age of thirteen.

PATIENT: The only thing that I remember is that I wouldn't dance for the life of me. Once my father was angry with my mother when she urged me to dance. He said, "Leave him alone, he has more important things to do." But my mother kept on saying that I "moved" so well with music. She wanted me to dance with her, but I refused point-blank, and she was disappointed.

THERAPIST: You seem to have a lot of feeling about "dancing," "praise" from your mother, and so on. We must look into all this.

The patient looked embarrassed but continued to give many details about his relations with his parents. He also mentioned that his mother wanted him to study in France so as not to be so far away from her. He said that deep inside he also preferred to study in Paris, being fascinated by that city, but decided to come to Boston instead for his college education at the urging of his father, who had studied in the United States. It was in Boston when he was about to get his BA degree that his symptoms appeared for the first time, as has already been mentioned.

Generally speaking, the therapist was less active in this first interview than is usual in STAPP because, as I mentioned already, the patient seemed to be more disturbed than other patients with obsessive-compulsive symptoms whom we had treated with this method. His illness seemed to be more serious, its onset was not of an acute nature, and his symptoms were more incapaciting, threatening to lead to complete paralysis.

It is of interest, however, that although he started at first to talk about his current academic difficulties, he quickly reverted to the conflicts with his parents, the focus of his STAPP.

SECOND INTERVIEW

The patient began this session by mentioning that he had visited his girlfriend, Susan, in Chicago and helped her write an essay without any difficulty. He was amazed that he was able to do this for her, while he had been unable to write a paper for himself. He also added, however, that when she started to thank him for his help, he became irritable because her attitude reminded him of his father's. He went on.

PATIENT: My relationship with my father, possibly because of beginning psychotherapy, as well as after a discussion that I had with a psychologist friend of mine who actually referred me to this clinic, is very much in my mind. I got irritated with Susan, as I told you, because her attitude of admiration was very much like my father's.

THERAPIST: Can you tell me more about this irritation at your father?

PATIENT: Well, it is not real irritation. It is more a feeling of vague annoyance. (*He proceeded to go into obsessive details about the differences in the meaning of the words "irritable" and "annoyed."*)

THERAPIST: (*interrupting*): You are going into all these subtle details to avoid looking at the parallel between Susan and your father?

PATIENT: It is interesting what you say, because Susan said to tell Dr. Sifneos that "I am an extension of my father."

THERAPIST: Hm.

PATIENT: Well, it is her attitude which also reminds me of my mother's, paying attention, trying to please me like my mother's attitude with my brother.

THERAPIST: Brother?

PATIENT: I meant to say father.

THERAPIST: Why did you make a slip of the tongue?

PATIENT: It is this kind of loving attention my father gets from my mother. She loves him romantically. She is loving, but unloved. She is lovable, yet my father does not reciprocate her love. Once he told me that he was "attached" to her. I thought, "Damn it, you are her husband. You owe her more than an attachment." (*with much feeling, pounding his fist on the table*)

THERAPIST: You are so irritated, almost angry.

PATIENT: Not then.

THERAPIST: Just now.

PATIENT: Now, yes, but when he told me I don't recall being annoyed.

THERAPIST: I meant that you were angry just now.

PATIENT: Yes, because he received her love, but he did not reciprocate it. Unreciprocated love.

THERAPIST: Are you jealous of your father?

PATIENT: . . . I don't understand. Jealous? I was not annoyed, as I told you.

THERAPIST: But you are now, and you just admitted it. Are you denying it?

PATIENT: Well, yes and no. It is all confusing. I don't understand. Jealous, you say?

THERAPIST: Please do not run away from your feelings. Let us recapitulate. You said that you were irritated with Susan because she
reminded you of your father's attitude. We also know that Susan's
expression of love reminds you of your mother's love for your
father, an unreciprocated love which makes you angry and, I add,
this is my word, possibly jealous. "After all, you are her husband," you said with great irritation. So when I ask you whether
you are jealous of your father you become confused, mixed up,
you don't understand. Now, what about this? Is my summary correct? Do you agree? No! Change it if you don't agree.

PATIENT: Well, if you want to call it "jealous."

THERAPIST: What do you call it?

PATIENT: Father does get all this attention from her which, yes, it
does irritate me at times but—(hesitating) but I also get attention
from my mother, of sorts. (smiling) You see there have been some
problems between my parents over the last few years . . . and
. . . you see—(hesitating)

THERAPIST: Go ahead.

PATIENT: My mother has been confiding to me, as I told you, she
needs me. (smiling)

THERAPIST: You smile.

PATIENT: So you see, I have been the center of attention from both
of my parents, but in entirely different ways. Now, as I mentioned, there have been big problems between them—my mother
gave me the impression that my father had recently become impotent with her.

THERAPIST: Gave you the impression?

PATIENT: Yes, in a roundabout way she insinuated that my father
was very upset about his sexual performance, but my mother
doesn't care. She is happy with and without sex. She is so easy-
going.

THERAPIST: So, can we hear more about being your mother's confi-
dant? I can see that the idea pleases you.

PATIENT: There was an episode many years ago when my father
wanted a divorce because he was in love with another woman,
but my mother wouldn't think of it. My father suspected that she
became pregnant with my brother so as just to make it impossible
for him to leave her. I think this also plays a role in his attitude

for my brother. He blames him for being the cause of his staying married.

THERAPIST: How do you feel abut all this?

PATIENT: Relieved to be able to talk about it, but also guilty. I would like to help both of my parents (*with much feeling*) because I love both of them very much.

THERAPIST: Yes, of course, and it is this love for both of them that makes the whole thing difficult. You have to choose between two people whom you love. It is quite a dilemma.

THIRD INTERVIEW

PATIENT: Am I supposed to be doing some thinking between sessions?

THERAPIST: Supposed? You are not supposed to be doing anything.

PATIENT: Maybe there is an area I should be talking about. (*He went on in detail for a while.*)

THERAPIST: You seem to be asking for direction today. We have agreed on a special focus to concentrate upon and to investigate. Have you forgotten what it was, or are you trying to get away from this important area because it makes you anxious?

PATIENT: Yes, of course! Thank you for reminding me.

THERAPIST: Why do you feel passive today?

PATIENT: I worked hard last time.

THERAPIST: You did, but you can work even harder today.

PATIENT: We talked about certain attitudes which I had for my parents. (*He again went into detail.*)

THERAPIST: Precisely, but you try to run away going into all these details.

PATIENT: We mentioned my feelings for Susan and my mother, and all these tales and confidences which she inundated me with.

THERAPIST: Inundated you? An interesting word!

PATIENT: It was like . . . I don't remember the term . . . The term that my behavior therapist used. . . . Oh, yes, "flooding." It was as if I were flooded by my mother's confidences. She pesters me and she keeps on pestering me. When Susan mothers me it irritates me in the same way. (*smiling*)

THERAPIST: Being pestered by both of them may irritate you, but you smile. Furthermore, your mother's confidences have a very special character; she came to you with her problems. I thought that you were pleased.

PATIENT: (sheepishly): It irritated me only if I had too much of it. It was embarrassing. I don't like to be flooded with it. It doesn't work.

THERAPIST: It seems that you emphasize the irritation, the negative features of your interaction with your mother. Is it to avoid the positive features? Tell me honestly, how did you feel when your mother confided in you some very important details about her relation with your father?

PATIENT: It didn't shock me.

THERAPIST: (*speaking slowing and emphasizing every word*): How did you feel when you heard all about your parents' sexual life? (*The therapist tries to pin him down with his anxiety-provoking confrontation.*)

PATIENT: . . . Hm . . . I don't know.

THERAPIST: What do you mean, you don't know?

PATIENT: I really don't know.

THERAPIST: Come on, now! Don't run away.

PATIENT: . . . I am at a loss. . . . This is a difficult area; rationally it—

THERAPIST: (*interrupting*): Don't rationalize and intellectualize in order to avoid this issue.

PATIENT: I reacted intensely.

THERAPIST: To what? Hearing about your father's impotence or your mother's sexual needs?

PATIENT: My mother was overdoing it, as I tried to tell you. I felt irritated to hear that my father did not love her, and that he did not get stimulated by her.

THERAPIST: So that's what the irritation is all about. Now, how did you feel about your mother's confiding all this to you, not about your irritation with your father?

PATIENT (*looking very tense*): I felt that I was a substitute.

THERAPIST: A substitute?

PATIENT: Yes! One night I remember I was asleep. My mother came to my room and woke me up. It was around one o'clock in the morning. She was in her nightgown. She looked very upset and told me that my father tried to have sex with her. At first she discouraged him, but later she felt arousal, but my father was impotent again.

THERAPIST: So how did you feel?

PATIENT: I told her that I didn't want to hear about it, but she insisted and said that if I were thirty years older, I would have made—(*hesitating*)—Well, she said, "If I had a man like you! You would have made a better husband for me." (*blinking*)

THERAPIST: And how did you feel?

PATIENT: Well . . . I felt flattered. She implied that I was better than my father.

THERAPIST: Implied! She spoke point-blank, and you call that "implied"! Furthermore she said more than that. She said that your father was not sexual and "implied"—yes you are right about the term—and implied that *you* were sexual.

PATIENT: . . . I felt ridiculous. I am not her husband!

THERAPIST: Ridiculous, eh? The same feeling which you experienced when your mother admired your "dancing movements"?

PATIENT: . . . I cannot think straight.

THERAPIST: What were your fantasies about being your mother's "thirty-year-older husband"?

PATIENT: You drive me out of my mind with your questions. I feel impotent intellectually.

THERAPIST: So, you identify with your father's impotence with an "intellectual impotence," to escape from your desires for your mother.

PATIENT: (*sighing as if he had not heard the above clarification*): Coming back to your question, my mother is beautiful but she is not my type. She always used to ask me if I thought that she was beautiful. I would say, "Yes, you are beautiful, but you are *not* my type."

THERAPIST: Now, you told me once what your mother looked like, but let's try again. What does your mother look like?

PATIENT: When she was young she was "fresh," but now she is fading away.

THERAPIST: But all these confidences took place when you were how old?

PATIENT: Oh, long ago, not recently, when I was thirteen or fourteen. My mother has a nice face, oval, not *very* beautiful. She has a very nice figure, tall, big-breasted, very "coquettish," but—

THERAPIST: And what does Susan look like?

PATIENT: Susan is less beautiful. She is very thin, almost flat-chested. She is also not my type.

THERAPIST: What is your type?

PATIENT: I have no type. . . . Your questions drive me up the wall.

THERAPIST: Yes, I know that they do, but time has come to your rescue. We must stop now!

By the end of this interview it is clear that the therapy is rapidly reaching its climax. Despite the patient's attempts to intellectualize and obsess as well as to run away from the anxiety-provoking confrontations and clarification of the therapist, he nevertheless is motivated to change. He stays within the specified focus and works hard at resolving the psychological conflicts which he is facing.

FOURTH INTERVIEW

The patient returned to Boston after a two-week Christmas vacation.

PATIENT: The last hour that we had was very difficult. But, first things first, I had a very dramatic episode with Susan. It probably had to do with our work here. We had a conflict. She pesters me and acts like a watchdog. She is so disciplined. She can catch me whenever she wants.

THERAPIST: Catch you at doing what?

PATIENT: (paying no attention): She is so smart and I am so attached to her, but she irritates me when she acts like a watchdog.

The therapist is caught in a dilemma. He wants to confront the patient with his identification with his father when he used the word "attached" to Susan in the same as his father was "attached" to his mother, which had made him angry. In addition, however, he is eager to hear about the dramatic episode and chooses to pursue that issue.

THERAPIST: What about Susan's being like a watchdog? Can we hear about what happened?

PATIENT: (Paying no attention, he talked at length about his vacation and started to give many irrelevant details about his airline reservations, etc.)

THERAPIST: (*interrupting him*): You go into all these details which serve the purpose simply to help you avoid your anxiety. Can we go back to the problem with Susan? (*This is a typical STAPP intervention, interfering with the patient's obsessive procrastinations.*)

PATIENT: OK. I had a short affair with someone for one week. It coincided with the beginning of my therapy here. When I visited Susan I told her about it, because she had always claimed that she didn't care, but when I told her, wow! She had quite a reaction. She was furious. She was hysterical. You see, I thought that she knew and I did not want to be caught lying. The worst thing is to lie and to be caught at it. So I told her. Well, you see, I don't regret having this brief affair. It was my "last fling." I need it. As I said, I don't regret it, but it was not a nice way to repay Susan, who has always been so supportive of me. Now I know that it is all over. I assure you of that.

THERAPIST: (*interrupting*): You don't have to use me as a father confessor. What is of interest is why did you have the affair as the "last fling," as you call it, and why did you have it just when you started your therapy?

The patient again went into details about how he was afraid that he would be caught lying and emphasized his love for Susan, and the fact that it was a "last fling," which he needed to have before discovering the reason for it during his therapy.

THERAPIST: I know all this, but why this great need which you mention so emphatically?

PATIENT: I like attractive women.

THERAPIST: Oh! You mean like your mother and Susan?

PATIENT: Hm.

THERAPIST: What did this woman—doesn't she have a name? What did she look like?

PATIENT: Muriel.

THERAPIST: What does Muriel look like?

PATIENT: Well, not like my mother, if that is what you have in mind.

THERAPIST: I asked you what she looked like. Leave what I have in mind to me.

PATIENT: (looking animated): She is a fellow student, very feminine, very attractive and coquettish.

THERAPIST: She doesn't remind you of anyone?

PATIENT: No.

THERAPIST: No?

PATIENT: (*smiling—giggling*): But now that you ask, she is coquettish like my mother. By God, I never saw this connection until this very minute. (*looking very surprised*)

THERAPIST: It does not surprise me in the least!

PATIENT: Oh, Dr. Sifneos, you do not have to be so sarcastic.

THERAPIST: I am not sarcastic in the slightest, but I did want you to see the connection with your mother. It had to come from you, however. The use of the word "coquettish" for both of them clinches it. In the same way as you used the word "pestering" about your mother and Susan. Now can you give me some more details about this brief affair?

PATIENT: This was the first and the last time. I want to reassure you. I love Susan and I want to marry her. I am in love. I was not in love with Muriel. I told her so and she understood. It was just a physical, a chemical attraction. (*He again tries to reassure the therapist by using the word "reassure" over and over about his love for Susan, and about the fact that his fling was his last one.*)

THERAPIST: You again seem to act as if you were confessing to a priest. I am not here to judge you. I simply asked you a question about this brief affair. I need no reassurance from you.

PATIENT: Muriel is very attractive. She is very dark. She is different from my mother.

THERAPIST: So, now you deny again the connection with your mother, when we had it a minute ago?

PATIENT: She is different, but she is very coquettish.

THERAPIST: And we know that your mother was and is very coquettish.

PATIENT: (*blushing*): Yes, this is true. (*looking very tired*) I told Muriel that I was in love with Susan. She was very understanding. I was confused. It even affected my sex drive at first. I couldn't have a solid erection, it would wilt away. I was impotent and then I couldn't control my orgasm. I ejaculated. I botched the whole thing. Muriel was very supportive as we tried again, and it was better and after a couple of days it was fine. The same thing had happened with Susan when we first met.

THERAPIST: Now, did you have this sexual problem because she reminded you of your mother or because you thought of your father?

PATIENT: No.

THERAPIST: What do you mean—no?

PATIENT: (remains silent)

THERAPIST: You are silent. Come on, now. Don't we know that your father had the exact same sexual problem with your mother as you had with Muriel?

PATIENT: (putting his hands on his face): Wow! This—this is very hard. You have given me quite a load of feeling. It is so confusing.

THERAPIST: This is true. This is difficult all right. This is the reason why we call this treatment "anxiety-provoking." But now it is time to stop.

This again was a very anxiety-producing interview. The ability to draw a parallel between Muriel and his mother as well as the patient's identification with the sexual impotence of his father brought the whole Oedipal focus into the open and gave rise to a great deal of affect. In a patient with an obsessive-compulsive personality structure where feelings were strongly defended by formidable defense mechanisms, this may be viewed as being an accomplishment.

Up to now this therapy clearly demonstrates the pattern of STAPP between two members of the same sex. It was safer for the patient to talk at first about his relations with women; now, however, he is faced with an even more difficult task. He has to talk abut his competitive feelings for his father, and men in general, and has to experience the same competitive feelings in his transference for the therapist.

FIFTH INTERVIEW

PATIENT: I felt very unsettled after our last interview. My eyelids were twitching for fifteen minutes after I left. When I was in the elevator I felt as if I had a facial tic. I thought, Oh boy, this treatment is getting to me. By the way this is exam time. Also, Susan and I got engaged last week and we plan to get married in Rome this summer.

THERAPIST: Congratulations.

PATIENT: Thank you.

THERAPIST: You announce three important things all at the same time. Which one shall we deal with first?

PATIENT: Well, about my anxiety. Susan wanted me to call you and ask you to give me some tranquilizing pills.

THERAPIST: I see.

PATIENT: I couldn't call you. I thought that it was antitherapeutic.

THERAPIST: I agree with you. If the therapy makes you anxious because you discuss all these problems with your parents, and if we gave you pills to decrease this anxiety, then the implications would be that you are weak, that you could not deal with it, and that we should drop discussing the subject that makes you anxious. In that case, we would be giving you a double message. Now, since you bring up an issue that has something to do between you and me, can we hear more about it?

The therapist takes advantage of the possibility to discuss the transference feelings which for all intents and purposes have not been clarified adequately as yet.

PATIENT: I didn't want any pills. I took two of my exams. I was tense but I am sure that I passed. It was not as bad as I had thought.

The patient proceeded to go into various details about his exams. The therapist, although interested to hear that he seemed to be dealing with the academic difficulties more effectively, was nevertheless sure that the patient was using this discussion as bait so as to avoid dealing with the transference feelings. He therefore decided to raise this issue again.

THERAPIST: Let's get back to discussing the feelings between us.

PATIENT: Yes, but there are some other points which I wanted to bring up about the exams.

THERAPIST: What about you and me?

PATIENT: You mean my feelings for you now?

THERAPIST: Yes.

PATIENT: Well, these are real issues, but I cannot see through them very clearly. I feel confused.

THERAPIST: Shall I repeat my questions once more?

PATIENT: (irritably): No. . . . You seem to have confidence that I can see through all this confusion. Yet—

THERAPIST: Yet?

PATIENT: Yet I feel that I can avoid some of your questions. It's a cat-and-mouse game but—well, I don't know if I can succeed to evade all your questions.

THERAPIST: So, there is competition going on between us and you feel that you may win. Furthermore, there is also this point of my having confidence in you. What does all this remind you of?

PATIENT: Vaguely . . . of my father.

THERAPIST: Vaguely! Come on, now!

PATIENT: Yes, but there are differences.

THERAPIST: In what way?

PATIENT: You are not unkind. You are not as rigid as he is. You are quick. You don't let me off the hook—well, maybe for a few seconds only. You pursue your points, but in a way this is what my father did. He pursued his points doggedly. You don't give me any rest. Your questions feel like daggers, but I also know that I feel pride when I can avoid them. Yet I know that you are trying to help me. Yes, your attitude reminds me of my father because he also wants to help me. It's all mixed up.

THERAPIST: So, there is clearly a connection between your feelings for your father and your feelings for me.

PATIENT: Yes, of course, but the differences are very important. You cut me off. You don't let me ramble all over the place. I am aware that this is one of my most successful techniques. (*He went into giving some details of how he was able to evade his father's questions and felt pride in having defeated him.*) You are more understanding; you give me credit without being ebullient like my father. In his pride about me he can never understand that I may also have some defects. . . . (*He looked as if he were on the verge of tears.*)

THERAPIST: You see that it is important to talk about your feelings here for me because it will help us to see what feelings of your belong to me and what feelings are displaced on me from other people, such as your father. As you can see, at first you resisted to do it and I had to press you, but now that you did, was it so bad?

PATIENT: No. I do feel much better now that it is all in the open.

This interview gave the therapist an opportunity to deal with the transference explicitly and once more to make a parent-transference link.

SIXTH INTERVIEW

Because of the midwinter vacation, the patient took a two-week trip to Italy for winter sports and a visit with his parents. The therapist, in anticipation, had in mind to recapitulate the work that had already been done, to consolidate what had been learned, but he soon found out that it was not necessary.

PATIENT: As you would expect, I also visited my parents after a beautiful week of skiing in the Alps. It was amazing to see my father exactly in the way that I have described him to you. I realized how much his attention is centered on me. I am his only delight. I felt pity for him because his only pleasure in life is my academic success. He was very upset to hear about my problems with my exam as I had anticipated, but this time it did not bother me so much because of all our work on it here. I know that being successful—(hesitating) even sexually successful, I would be better than my father.

THERAPIST: And if you are "his only delight," then—

PATIENT: I defeat him. He has nothing to live for. He withers away and dies.

THERAPIST: So you must fail in order to keep your father alive. Furthermore, any success in chess, in dancing, academically, becomes an instrument which eliminates your father whom you love and whom you don't want to kill. So failure becomes inevitable.

PATIENT: Indeed.

THERAPIST: If you defeat your father even in the sexual area with your mother, then not only you defeat him but you also humiliate him and this you cannot do, so you become impotent with the coquettish Muriel, who reminds you of your mother, as a way out.

PATIENT: You put it so clearly. It makes me cringe.

THERAPIST: Of course, but there are two advantages to all this. Number one, it is all in the open, not hidden away and forcing you to run away from it. Second, yours is a neurotic solution. There is a way out of it. But first things first. How were things in Rome with your mother?

PATIENT: (The patient in his usual way proceeded to go on about a great number of details without answering the question.)

THERAPIST: (*interrupting*): I asked you a simple question and there you go again trying to avoid it. Is this your way of defeating me also? Now, how did you get along with your mother?

PATIENT: I had a date with one of my ex-girlfriends—mind you, no fling or sex or anything. We are friends and we had dinner together and I brought her to my parents' home afterwards. In any case, my mother came in while we were sitting on the couch drinking cognac, but she apologized for interrupting us and she left. The next day my mother asked me a lot of questions. Was Beatrice attractive to me; did I find her more beautiful than her? She acted very coquettish as she asked these questions and kept on pestering me, but I remembered what we had discussed here, and so I did not feel as excited and flattered as I used to be. Finally, when my mother started asking me about my sexual relations with Susan, I told her that she was nosy, that she was meddling into my private affairs, that it was none of her business, and that her attitude was uncalled for.

THERAPIST: Well, our work seems to be paying dividends.

PATIENT: Yes, indeed.

THERAPIST: It does not have to be the other extreme, however. What I mean is that you don't have to be nasty at your mother's expense.

PATIENT: No. No. I know what you mean. Yes, my mother's feelings were hurt a bit, but after I discussed my need for independence with her, she was very understanding.

THERAPIST: I am glad to hear it.

This episode was the first indication to the therapist that a tangible evidence of change in the patient's behavior was taking place. He dealt with his mother realistically. Rather than answer her questions because of his attraction for her coquettishness, he stands up to her about his relations with Susan and is able to draw the line with her. Generally speaking, the first part of the Oedipal focus—namely, his relations with women in general and his sexual attraction for his mother in particular—has been dealt with adequately. The remaining work to be done has to do with the resolution of his feelings for his "defeated father" as well as his transference feelings for his male therapist.

It is of interest that the patient brings the subject up during the next interview.

SEVENTH INTERVIEW

PATIENT: I lost my wallet twice during the past week, and four times during the last few months. I also had some sexual problems with Susan, who was here visiting me. It was not too bad, but sex was not as good as it used to be. I seemed to be losing my erections off and on. . . . I was an "absentminded professor."

THERAPIST: Again you seem to be talking about two different things at the same time. Now who called you an "absentminded professor"?

PATIENT: My mother. She used to call me that and would joke about it.

THERAPIST: After announcing that your attitude for your mother had changed, are you acting like an absentminded professor in order to please her? . . . Now what is the significance of losing your wallet? What does a wallet represent?

PATIENT: Well, a wallet represents one's own capabilities and one's power.

THERAPIST: What kind of power?

PATIENT: Power, political power, intellectual power, academic power, sexual power.

THERAPIST: And?

PATIENT: That is all.

THERAPIST: I am intrigued that you mention all kinds of power, yet you do not include the most obvious, financial power. After all, a wallet is a place where one keeps one's money!

PATIENT: I know that, but clearly financial power is not what I had in mind.

THERAPIST: So if you lose this intellectual, sexual power, you become powerless, and isn't that what happened with Susan? You say that you were semi-impotent. You lost your sexual power?

Although the therapist wanted to have more association about the meaning of the wallet, he saw an opportunity to connect the patient's sexual and academic problems. This may have been premature and therefore a mistake.

PATIENT: As you know, we talked about all this already. What comes to my mind is my mother confiding in me about their sexual difficulties.

THERAPIST: Precisely. So why do you throw your sexual power away by losing your wallet, as well as in reality with Susan?

PATIENT: You are like my father. You pursue the same points over and over.

THERAPIST: No, I am not. *You* are like your father when you have your sexual impotence. We have been through all this. Yes. Your competitions with him, your defeat of him, and your identification with him.

PATIENT: . . . In a peculiar way, as you were talking, I thought that you were mad at me. I don't know. Your facial expressions reminded me of my father's when he got angry at my brother.

THERAPIST: Of course! This is a different picture that we have of your father. The angry, rigid father. What would your father think if he were to know that you were flirting with his coquettish wife? We have seen that one possibility is that he would have felt defeated by you, but is that the only one? Is it also possible that your father may not like the idea at all, and that he may get mad at you as you have just thought that I was angry with you?

PATIENT: It is possible but unlikely.

THERAPIST: If he were, what comes to your mind?

PATIENT: Castration comes to my mind.

THERAPIST: Do you say this because you think that this is what I want to hear? I don't want to hear anything except what goes through *your* mind.

PATIENT: No. You don't understand. (*getting irritated*) I really meant it when I said castration.

THERAPIST: And what does castration then imply?

PATIENT: I don't know what you mean.

THERAPIST: I mean exactly what I mean. What is a castrated man?

PATIENT: Someone who cannot perform or enjoy.

THERAPIST: Yes, indeed. So, being castrated is a perfect way out.

PATIENT: Way out? Out of what?

THERAPIST: Out of the trouble that he has gotten himself into.

PATIENT: I don't follow you.

THERAPIST: You don't because you are resisting. If you cannot perform sexually, if you lose your sexual power, if you are a "castrated" man," then your father has nothing to fear from you. There is no competition between the two of you. Your father can relax. He doesn't have to be jealouos about your flirtations with your mother. He doesn't have to get mad. How can he get mad at an impotent, sexually powerless, castrated man? This is "the way out." You castrate yourself. You become impotent. You lose your sexual powers, your wallet; so you throw your penis away, in self-defense, to protect yourself, to avoid any punishment.

PATIENT: . . . He did have quite a temper at times. . . . But you know I feel very queer now. This whole thing makes me feel much better. It makes all the sense to me. Things are beginning to click. (*smiling broadly*)

THERAPIST: Now that the sexual area is very clear, let us not forget that there is another aspect to your power, this "intellectual power" of yours. Isn't this what happens when you are unable to prepare yourself for your exams or to finish your papers?

PATIENT: It is interesting because what you say reminds me of a fellow student, a girl who was married and was interested in me. I liked her and I was attracted to her, but I started feeling apprehensive, thinking that if I saw her too often she would take too much of my time. So I avoided her in order to study for my exams, *but I couldn't study*. As you say, I gave up my intellectual power because I was attracted to her. I was attracted to an attached woman. It is so fantastic! I can see things now so much more clearly.

He continued giving a variety of examples about his anxieties and fears of his examinations.

This session was very significant because the patient was able to see that there was a connection between his sexual and his academic difficulties, which were the complaints that brought him to the clinic.

EIGHTH INTERVIEW

He came 8 minutes late for this interview. This was surprising because he had always been extremely punctual, arriving at the clinic at least 15 minutes before his appointment time.

PATIENT: I am sorry to be late, but I noticed lately that I am not as well prepared as I used to be.

THERAPIST: Are you saying that you are more relaxed than what you used to be?

PATIENT: Yes, in a way. For example, you won't believe it but I managed to turn in a paper on time.

THERAPIST: I do believe you!

PATIENT: It was on the last minute, but I did it nevertheless. (*He went on giving some details in his usual way.*)

THERAPIST: You go on and on with these details. Is it a way of undoing your success in managing to turn in your paper on time?

PATIENT (*smiling*): No, no. (*From then on the patient started to talk about one of his professors.*) By the way, I got an A in my latest quiz. This paper that I mentioned was a good one, not because my professor told me so but rather because I think so. I had the thought that I might send it to my father. I had that feeling of competition with him, but also I know that I am like him.

THERAPIST: Yes, you are—at least sexually.

PATIENT (*laughing*): You know, I had no sexual difficulties with Susan whatsoever, and this is surprising because off and on I had some problems in the past.

THERAPIST: Let me recapitulate where we are. We have worked hard on this problem and our work seems to have paid off. Your feelings for your mother, it seems, have been clarified. There are a few aspects of your relationships with men in authority, such as your professors, and of course with your father, which have to be scrutinized before we end this therapy. After all, don't forget that your feelings here for me reflect some of these conflicts which you have with men in general.

Although the patient seemed to agree, his associations to this clarification pointed in the opposite direction. He immediately started to talk about his courses in his usual detached way, but rarely did he make any reference to his feelings for his professors. Despite the thearpist's efforts he managed to slip away.

It seemed obvious to the therapist at the end of this interview that his tendency to undo his success was associated with some unresolved transference issues which had to be worked through before termination of his treatment.

NINTH INTERVIEW

PATIENT: Let me give you a list of the various courses and papers which I shall have to take and to write next semester—

THERAPIST: (*interrupting*): Is this list that you plan to give me a way of avoiding to discuss your feelings for your father as well as your feelings for me?

PATIENT: (*paying no attention*): There is a course given by one of my teachers.

THERAPIST: A nameless one!

PATIENT: Professor Y.

THERAPIST: What are your feelings for him?

PATIENT: I pity him because he is driven by his wife.

THERAPIST: Familiar, don't you think?

PATIENT: (*hesitating*): Well, if you mean that I have pity for him in the same way that I felt pity for my father, yes, this is true.

THERAPIST: Now what about this "driving wife"?

PATIENT: She is an attractive middle-aged woman. I suspect that there is a lot of trouble between them. During one cocktail party she spent much time talking to me.

THERAPIST: I see!

PATIENT: I feel irritated by Professor Y and by your attitude. Both of you tend to interrupt without saying anything of significance or of substance.

THERAPIST: (*ignoring the negative transference, persists in his inquiry about the professor's wife*): What about his wife?

PATIENT: You always want to hear about these women. (*irritably*) She is not like my mother.

THERAPIST: Your anger at me makes you unable to hear what I asked. I did not mention your mother.

PATIENT: Yes, I know. Professor Y irritates me because he always says that I know more than he does, just like my father. Are you satisfied?

THERAPIST: Shall we talk about your anger at me today?

PATIENT: You make me feel insecure with your questions.

THERAPIST: I thought that they were of no "significance or substance."

PATIENT: I am angry because I feel pressed by you to pursue these issues with my father. I thought that we have talked all about those.

THERAPIST: The fact that you are annoyed means that we haven't done our work completely.

PATIENT: You know that I fit into some kind of a pattern and you drive hard at it, but I know that—(*smiling*)

THERAPIST: That you can defeat me also, and fail in your treatment?

PATIENT: (*flabbergasted*): Oh, no, no. You know that it is not true what you say. You know that I work hard here.

THERAPIST: You do up to a certain point, but when the going is getting rough you try to run away with your obsessive details and all your familiar maneuvers. I understand it, but I won't let you escape.

PATIENT: I—

THERAPIST: How do you feel right now?

PATIENT: I feel unsettled.

THERAPIST: So, let us hear about your unsettled feelings as a result of your relations to me.

PATIENT: I have said it already. You are quick and you drive hard at your points. You make me feel irritable and anxious. Today you remind me very much of Professor Y.

THERAPIST: Professor Y and your father. You become annoyed when I asked you about Professor Y's wife. Is there also a woman between us?

PATIENT: I know—(*hesitating*) I don't know any women who know you.

THERAPIST: Why did you hesitate?

PATIENT: The other day I happened to see you in your old car at Harvard Square.

THERAPIST: What about my old car?

PATIENT: Well, I thought that you would be driving a better car. Even my car is better than yours.

THERAPIST: So, there is competition in the area of cars and you think that you win. Anything else about seeing me in my old car at Harvard Square?

PATIENT: No.

THERAPIST: No?

PATIENT: Your wife was also inside.

THERAPIST: So, there is a woman between us! Can we hear more about it?

PATIENT: There you go again. You make a mountain out of a molehill!

THERAPIST: Come on, now—

PATIENT: (*interrupting*): She did look a bit like Professor Y's wife, but she looked much younger. She looked very "fresh."

THERAPIST: You mean like your mother?

PATIENT: By God! It is true. I never thought of it.

The therapist's use of the exact words which are used by the patients whenever making a confrontation, clarification, or an interpretation always makes an impact on them. Such words as "fresh," "coquettish," "pestered" have been used by the patient and the therapist in the context of STAPP.

THERAPIST: You feel irritable with me in the same way that you felt with Professor Y and your father. Do you want to flirt also with my wife?
PATIENT: (*blushing*): It is interesting. How did you know? The thought had just crossed my mind when I saw you at Harvard Square. I thought, "Maybe I'll meet her at a Harvard cocktail party." You read my mind!
THERAPIST: I am not a magician. It is so obvious!
PATIENT: That was not all. You see, I thought that you would be called to the hospital on an emergency so I would offer to drive Mrs. Sifneos to your home.
THERAPIST: Don't you think that now we have all the pieces of your jigsaw puzzle put neatly in place?
PATIENT: Yes, I think so.

At this point the therapist recapitulated the issues which had already been dealt with in the therapy, and ended by suggesting that it was time to think about termination. Again in this interview the transference feelings were linked with parents or parent substitutes. The competitive feelings which predominate between patients and therapists of the same sex at the latter stages of STAPP were also dealt with appropriately.

TENTH INTERVIEW

PATIENT: It was quite a week! Susan was here all week. I was very much aware of our discussions here. We had a good dinner with Susan but I felt tired. Susan asked me if I wanted to have intercourse, but I said that I was exhausted and said, "Maybe tomorrow." I went to bed. She stayed and watched TV. When she came to bed she woke me up. She was wearing her nightgown but she took it off and again asked me to have sex with her. She looked very attractive, but I couldn't have an erection.

THERAPIST: So you identified again with your father.

PATIENT: I was tired, as I told you.

THERAPIST: Yes, but it is identical with the time when your mother came to your room in her nightgown and told you about your father's impotence and her wish for you to have been thirty years older to be her husband. (*The therapist proceeded to recapitulate the patient's relations with his parents in some detail.*)

PATIENT: It is true, but there was a redeeming feature about it all. I thought of this episode with my mother, maybe not as explicitly as you put it, but I did, and I decided to try to have sexual intercourse as a way to test my therapy, and you know it worked. I thought, "Susan is Susan and my mother is my mother." I felt proud of myself.

THERAPIST: You deserve to feel proud. You worked hard in your therapy and you solved your problem. You see, it is fairly simple. Once one has the courage to look at the truth, painful as it may be, one can achieve anything he wants.

PATIENT: I have been feeling good lately.

THERAPIST: When shall we stop?

PATIENT: Oh? Not yet. I like this treatment.

THERAPIST: I know that you do, but we have achieved what we had set up to do. As you know, we decided that it was going to be short-term. Let me see, this is our tenth session. It doesn't mean that it has to be our last one, but let us decide how many more you would need to round things up. When are your exams?

PATIENT: In a few weeks.

THERAPIST: How do you feel about the prospect?

PATIENT: Confident.

THERAPIST: OK. Then maybe we can have three more hours and then end.

PATIENT: All right.

During the next two interviews most of the time was spent in summarizing and consolidating what had been accomplished. The patient emphasized how much he had learned about himself in reference to his feelings for his parents. He said that he was much more relaxed about the prospect of his exams. He stressed the fact that he understood and was not upset by his forbidden wishes for his mother. Furthermore, he felt much less pity and very little in the way of competitive feelings for his father and Professor Y. His relations with Susan, both emotional and sexual, were fine, and he added sheepishly, "I don't feel irritated at you anymore, Dr. Sifneos."

THIRTEENTH INTERVIEW

PATIENT: I had a quiz two days ago. I did well. I'll get an A minus or even an A, but this is a minor issue. I still procrastinate about studying, although it is much less than it ued to be. It has become a minor issue.

THERAPIST: Minor issue?

PATIENT: As we have decided, the major part of our work had to do with my feelings for my parents, and as we have been discussing the last few weeks, in this area I have a much better understanding.

THERAPIST: In retrospect, which interview stands out in your memory?

PATIENT: It is difficult to say. There were so many which were important, but I think the one when I discussed the loss of my wallet, as well as the one about your wife and my competition with you, were the highlights of this treatment.

THERAPIST: I agree.

PATIENT: There is also another change. I can get a $6000 grant to cover some of my expenses and do some teaching. In this way I won't have to depend on my father financially. It makes me feel independent!

THERAPIST: So, now what are your plans?

PATIENT: As you know, Susan and I will be getting married this summer in Rome. She is also graduating from college. I look forward to our married life. I realize that I displaced a lot of my feelings from my parents onto Susan. This was unfair. I am aware of this now and our relationship is better than ever. I know what feelings belong to what people.

The rest of the hour was uneventful. At the end he said:

PATIENT: This treatment was difficult, but the dividends are impressive.

THERAPIST: You talk like a successful businessman.

PATIENT: (*laughing*): I feel I have achieved a great deal.

THERAPIST: Yes, you have.

PATIENT: With your help.

THERAPIST: Yes.

PATIENT: Good-bye and thank you.

THERAPIST: You are very welcome indeed.

FOLLOW-UP INTERVIEW

The patient was seen by the therapist and by an independent evaluator one and one-half years after the end of his therapy. He missed his one-year follow-up interview because he had returned to Italy.

The two interviews were essentially identical. In terms of the criteria for outcome, this is what he had to say:

He felt that in general he was doing well and that his symptoms, namely, his academic difficulties, were much better. He had passed all his courses, having worked quite hard, and had obtained his degree. He said that during his exams he felt anxious, "like everybody else." When asked about his grades, he sheepishly answered that he did "very, very well" and that he got the best grades. Laughing, he added, "I guess I fooled my professor." In reference to his therapy he said he felt in retrospect that it was easy to see and accept the truth of what had transpired.

EVALUATOR: What about your feelings for your parents?

PATIENT: I recognized the intensity of my feelings for both my father and mother during my therapy, which I accept now much more easily than I did at the time.

EVALUATOR: What about your feelings for your father?

PATIENT: I felt pity for him. The clarification of my competitive feelings for him was very vivid and was very helpful. When I saw my father I felt relaxed, more distant. My feelings cooled off.

EVALUATOR: What about your mother?

PATIENT: I had felt resentful of my mother's "coquettishness," but also a great deal of attraction. My therapy helped me change my relationship with my mother. I was able to pinpoint my feelings for both of my parents. This resulted in a marked change for the better.

EVALUATOR: What about your girlfriend?

PATIENT: We have been married for one year. It was a wonderful year. Susan wants a child and we are working at it. There have been no sexual difficulties between us. The impotence has disappeared.

The scoring for the follow-up interviews has already been discussed. Scores fo 11 to 14 denote "recovery," 7 to 11 "much better," 3 to 7 "little better," 3 to 1 "unchanged."

This is how the independent evaluator rated the patient on the eight outcome criteria and the specific internal predisposition (SIP):

```
Symptoms
    Psychological          6)
                             ) = 6.5
    Physical               7)
Interpersonal relations
    With mother            6)
    With father            6) = 6
    With wife              6)
Self-understanding         6
    Problem solving        5
    New learning           6
    Self-esteem            5
    Work performance       5
    New attitudes          6   _____
        Total                  45.5 ÷ 8 = 5.68
SIP                        5            5.00
        Total                         10.68
```

Thus a score of 10.68 denotes that the patient was considered too be in the upper limits of the "much better" category.

The patient was also seen four and one-half years later for a second follow-up interview. He had been teaching at the business school of a well-known university for one and a half years. He had obtained his teaching appointment because of his superior performance and the excellent recommendations of his professor. His academic problem had disappeared. He stated that he had no difficulties in writing or reading. There were no sexual problems. Relations with his wife, father, and mother were fine. He emphasized and related in detail what he had learned in his therapy and that he was utilizing this knowledge in his everyday life, particularly in his ability to understand the psychological difficulties of his students, which had similarities to his own.

He was scored as follows:

Symptoms
Psychological	6)	
		) = 6.5
Physical	7)	
Interpersonal relations		
With father	7)	
With mother	6) = 6.6	
With wife	7)	
Self-understanding	6	
Problem solving	6	
New learning	7	
Self-esteem	6	
Work performance	6	
New attitudes	6	
	50.1 ÷ 8 = 6.26	
SIP	6	6.00
Total		12.26

Thus a score of 12.26 placed the patient in the "recovered" category.

In addition, during this follow-up interview the patient was shown the seventh videotape interview, which dealt with the loss of his wallet. His first remark was the following: "Oh, look at me. I am so Italian! I use my hands and my arms to make my points. I gesticulate so much. I am exactly like my father!"

Then he went on: "I was so different from what I am today. Look at me discussing all this 'power' business. I knew that I was resisting and I did not want to hear what was being said, yet I knew so well that it was true. What is of interest to me is that now it all looks so unimportant, so trivial. I feel a bit embarrassed for having been so neurotic!''

References

Adler, B., & Meyerson, P. (Eds.). *Confrontation in psychotherapy*, New York: Science House, 1973.

Alexander, F. Psychoanalytic contributions to short-term psychotherapy. In L. R. Wolberg (Ed.), *Short-term psychotherapy*. New York: Grune & Stratton, 1965, p. 84.

Alexander, F., & French, T. *Psychoanalytic psychotherapy*. New York: Ronald Press, 1946.

Barten, H. H. *Brief therapies*. New York: Behavioral Publications, 1971.

Bellak, L., & Small, L. *Emergency therapy and brief psychotherapy*. New York: Grune & Stratton, 1965.

Brusset, B. *De la psychotherapie à durée limitée et de la technique de evaluation et possibilités de changement*. Symposium sur psychothérapies analytiques brèves, Lausanne, June 22–25, 1983.

Davanloo, H. *Basic principles and techniques in a short-term dynamic psychotherapy*. New York: Spectrum Publications, 1978.

Davanloo, H. (Ed.). *Proceedings of the first and second international symposia for short-term dynamic psychotherapy*. In preparation.

Eitinger, L., & Heiberg, A. Psychotherapeutic problems: Research and plans at the Psychiatric Department, University of Oslo. In T. Mogstad & F. Magnussen (Eds.), *What is psychotherapy?* Basel, Switzerland: S. Karger, 1975.

Ferenczi, S. *Further contributions to the theory and technique of psychoanalysis*. London: Hogarth Press, 1926.

Ferenczi, S., & Rank, O. *The development of psychoanalysis*. New York: Nervous and Mental Disease Publishing, 1925.

Gillieron, E. *Au confins de la psychanalyse*. Paris: Payot, 1983.

Glover, E. *The technique of psychoanalysis*. New York: International Universities Press, 1955.

Gray, S. H. The resolution of the Oedipus complex in women. *Journal of the Philadelphia Association of Psychoanalysis*, 1976, 3, 103–111.

Guyotat, J. *Interventions psychothérapeutiques brèves focalization sur le lieu de filation*. Symposium sur psychothérapies analytiques brèves, Lausanne, June 22–25, 1983.

Horowitz, M. *Personality styles and brief psychotherapy*. New York: Basic Books, 1984.

Husby, R. A five year follow up of 36 neurotic patients. *Psychotherapy and Psychosomatics*, 1985, *43*, 17–23. (a)

Husby, R. Comparison of recorded changes in 33 neurotic patients 2 and 5 years after end of treatment. *Psychotherapy and Psychosomatics*, 1985, *43*, 23–28. (b)

Husby, R. Short-term dynamic psychotherapy IV. *Psychotherapy and Psychosomatics*, 1985, *43*, 28–32. (c)

Leeman, C. Outcome criteria in psychotherapy research. In T. Mogstad & F. Magnussen (Eds.), *What is psychotherapy?* Basel, Switzerland: S. Karger, 1975.

Malan, D. H. *The frontier of brief psychotherapy*. New York: Plenum Medical Books, 1976. (a)

Malan, D. H. *A study of brief psychotherapy*. New York: Plenum Rosetta Medical Publications, 1976. (b)

Malan, D. H. *Toward the validation of dynamic psychotherapy*. New York: Plenum Medical Books, 1976. (c)

Malan, D. H., Heath, E. S., Bacal, I., & Balfour, H. G. Psychodynamic changes in untreated neurotic patients. *Archives of General Psychiatry*, 1975, *32*, 110–127.

Mann, D. *Time limited psychotherapy*. Cambridge, Mass.: Harvard University Press, 1973.

Marty, P., de M'Uzan, M., & David, C. *L'investigation psychomatique*. Paris: Presses Universitaires de France, 1963.

McGuire, M. The process of short-term insight psychotherapy, I. *Journal of Nervous and Mental Disease*, 1965, *141*, 93–97. (a)

McGuire, M. The process of short-term insight psychotherapy. II. *Journal of Nervous and Mental Disease*, 1965, *141*, 219–223. (b)

McGuire, M. The instruction nature of short-term insight psychotherapy. *American Journal of Psychiatry*, 1968, *22*, 218–232.

McGuire, M., & Sifneos, P. E. Problems solving methods in psychotherapy. *Psychiatric Quarterly*, 1970, *44*, 667–674.

Montgrain, N. *Les effects thérapeutiques de construire une théorie sur soi*. Symposium sur psychothérapies analytiques brèves, Lausanne, June 22–25, 1983.

Nemiah, J. C. Alexithymia—Theoretical considerations. *Psychotherapy and Psychosomatics*, 1977, *28*, 199–206.

Nemiah, J. C., & Sifneos, P. E. Affect and fantasy in patients with psychosomatic disorders. In O. Hill (Ed.), *Modern trends in psychosomatic medicine*. London: Butterworths, 1970.

Porter, R. (Ed.). *The role of learning in psychotherapy*. London: J. and A. Churchill, 1968.

Schneider, P. *Propédeutique d'une psychothérapie*. Paris: Payot, 1976.

Shipko, S. Alexithymia and somatization. *Psychotherapy and Psychosomatics*, 1982, *37*, 193–201.

Sifneos, P. E. Dynamic psychotherapy in a psychiatric clinic. In I. Masserman (Ed.), *Current psychiatric therapies*. New York: Grune & Stratton, 1961, pp. 168–175.

Sifneos, P. E. Seven years' experience with short-term dynamic psychotherapy (Paper presented at the Sixth International Congress of Psychotherapy, London, 1964). In M. Pines & T. Spoerri (Ed.), *Psychotherapy and psychosomatics: Selected lecturers*. Basel and New York: S. Karger, 1965.

Sifneos, P. E. Psychoanalytically oriented short-term dynamic or anxiety-provoking psychotherapy for mild obsessional neuroses. *Psychiatric Quarterly*, 1966, *40*, 271–282.

Sifneos, P. E. Two different kinds of psychotherapy of short duration. *American Journal of Psychiatry*, 1967, *123*, 1069–1074.

Sifneos, P. E. Learning to solve emotional problems: A controlled study of short-term dynamic psychotherapy. In R. Porter (Ed.), *The role of learning in psychotherapy*. London: J. and A. Churchill, 1968. (a)

Sifneos, P. E. The motivational process. *Psychiatric Quarterly*, 1968, *42*, 271–279. (b)

Sifneos, P. E. Change in patient's motivation for psychotherapy. *American Journal of Psychiatry*, 1971, *128*, 718–722.

Sifneos, P. E. *Short-term psychotherapy and emotional crisis*. Cambridge, Mass.: Harvard University Press, 1972.

Sifneos, P. E. An overview of a psychiatric clinic population. *American Journal of Psychiatry*, 1973, *130*, 1032–1036.

Sifneos, P. E. Videotape: An educational and research tool for short-term psychotherapy. In H. Froshaug, D. Jeuback, & I. Ravnsborg (Ed.), *Visjon og vilje*. Oslo: Fabritius, 1975. (a)

Sifneos, P. E. Criteria for psychotherapeutic outcome. *Psychotherapy and Psychosomatics*. 1975, *26*, 49–58. (b)

Sifneos, P. E. Motivation for change: A prognostic guide for successful psychotherapy. *Psychotherapy and psychosomatics*, 1978, *29*, 293–298.

Sifneos, P. E. The current status of individual short-term dynamic psychotherapy and its future: An overview. *American Journal of Psychotherapy*, 1984, *37*(4).

Sifneos, P. E. Short-term dynamic psychotherapy of phobic and mildly obsessive-compulsive patients. *American Journal of Psychotherapy*, 1985, *39*(3).

Sifneos, P. E., Apfel-Saritz, R., & Frankel, F. The phenomenon of alexithymia. *Psychotherapy and Psychosomatics*, 1977, *28*, 47–57.

Strupp, H. H. & Binder, J. L. *Psychotherapy in a new key: A guide to time-limited psychotherapy*. New York: Basic, 1985.

Strupp, H. H., & Hadley, S. W. A tripartite model of mental health and therapeutic outcomes, with special reference to negative effects in psychotherapy. *American Psychologist*, 1977, *32*, 187–196.

Taylor, J. G. Alexithymia concept measurement and implications for treatment. *American Journal of Psychiatry*, 1984, *141*, 725–732.

Index

Printed in the United Kingdom
by Lightning Source UK Ltd.
120292UK00005BB/13